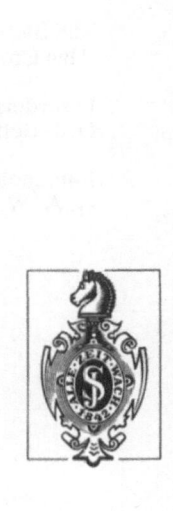

 The Bloomsbury Series in Clinical Science

HERPES SIMPLEX VIRUS

Adrian Mindel

With 51 Figures

Springer-Verlag
London Berlin Heidelberg New York
Paris Tokyo

Adrian Mindel, MB, BCh, MSc, MRCP
Senior Lecturer and Honorary Consultant in Genito-Urinary
Medicine, Academic Department of Genito-Urinary Medicine,
University College and Middlesex School of Medicine, James
Pringle House, The Middlesex Hospital, London W1N 8AA, UK

Series Editor

Jack Tinker, BSc, FRCS, FRCP, DIC
Director, Intensive Therapy Unit, The Middlesex Hospital,
London W1N 8AA, UK

Cover illustrations: background – Fig. 7.1c; foreground upper –
Fig. 7.4; foreground lower – Fig. 4.13.

British Library Cataloguing-in-Publication Data
Mindel, Adrian, 1949–
    Herpes simplex virus.
    1. Man. Herpes simplex
    I. Title II. Series
    616.5′2

Library of Congress Cataloging-in-Publication Data
Mindel, Adrian, 1949–
        Herpes simplex virus/Adrian Mindel.
        p. cm. — (The Bloomsbury series in clinical science)
        Bibliography: p.
        Includes index.

    ISBN-13: 978-1-4471-1685-1   e-ISBN-13: 978-1-4471-1683-7

    DOI: 10.1007/978-1-4471-1683-7

        1. Herpes simplex. 2. Herpes simplex virus. I. Title.
    II. Series.
    RC147.H6M56 1989
    616.9′25—dc19
    89–30659

Typeset by Goodfellow & Egan Limited, Cambridge

2128/3916-543210–Printed on acid-free paper

Series Editor's Foreword

Herpes Simplex Virus is the fifth monograph to be published in the Bloomsbury Series of Clinical Science. It provides an authoritative review of the key issues related to this common clinical problem. The characteristics of the virus, its epidemiology and the diagnosis and management of the various forms of infection are all considered.

Adrian Mindel is an international authority on this subject; he joined the Academic Department of Genito-urinary Medicine at the Middlesex Hospital in 1980 and has been actively involved in HSV research since that time. His major research interests include the epidemiology and treatment of genital herpes, the epidemiology of neo-natal herpes and the many and varied features of HSV infections in immuno-compromised patients.

The continuing aim of the Bloomsbury Series is to identify the growing areas of clinical research and relate these to current and future medical practice. In *Herpes Simplex Virus* such aspirations have been successfully achieved.

London, May 1989   Jack Tinker

Preface

There has been considerable interest in herpes simplex viruses (HSV) over recent years. Amongst the many reasons for this are the introduction of safe and efficacious therapy, the recognition that HSV may cause life-threatening infections in neonates and immunocompromised patients, the observation that genital herpes is one of the commonest viral sexually transmitted diseases and the possible association of HSV with cervical cancer.

Whilst it is now well established that HSV is often subclinical and that the virus establishes latency, our understanding of the natural history, pathogenesis and pathology of HSV infections is still somewhat patchy. The introduction of type-specific serological assays and the numerous advancements in molecular biology are now helping to unravel these complex issues.

This monograph is an attempt to bring together the clinical, epidemiological, immunological, pathological and virological aspects of HSV infections. It is written from a clinical perspective and therefore clinical features, diagnosis and treatment constitute the majority of the book. The sections on Virology, Immunology, Epidemiology, Pathology and Pathogenesis are relatively brief but I believe essential for a complete understanding of HSV infection.

November 1988   A.M.

Acknowledgements

I would like to thank Dr David Katz and Professor John Pattison for their help and advice, Stuart Nightingale and Angela Scott for their assistance with the preparation of the figures, Michael Jackson without whose persistence and persuasion this project would never have come to fruition, Katerina Ayres for typing the manuscript, my two Research Nurses, Orla Carney and Anna Faherty, for their help in the conduct of clinical studies, and finally all the patients who have participated in clinical studies at the Middlesex Hospital over the last eight years, without whose help none of this would have been possible.

Contents

Contents

Chapter 1

Virology and Immunology

Introduction

There are two herpes simplex viruses (HSV) designated HSV 1 and HSV 2. Although the two viruses are morphologically identical and have approximately 50% DNA similarity, there are a number of biological, biochemical, genomic and clinical differences between them. These are summarised in Table 1.1. The clinical differences will be highlighted in subsequent chapters, but here I will cover the basic virology and immunology of HSV infection.

Table 1.1. Comparison between HSV 1 and HSV 2

	HSV 1	HSV 2
Biological differences		
Replication in chick embryos	Poor	Form plaques
Sensitivity to BVDU	Sensitive	Insensitive
Neurovirulence in mice	+	+++
Livers of infected mice	Microscopic lesions	Macroscopic lesions
EM of infected cells	−	Microtubular structures
Biochemical differences		
DNA guanine + cytosine content (mole %)	67	69
Genomic differences	~ 50% DNA sequence similarity	
Clinical differences		
Oral infection	+++	+
Genital infection	+	+++
Eye infection	++	+
Brain infection	++	+
Neonatal infection	+	++
Disseminated infection	+	+

EM, electron microsopy; + etc., degree of reaction; BVDU, bromovinyl deoxyuridine.

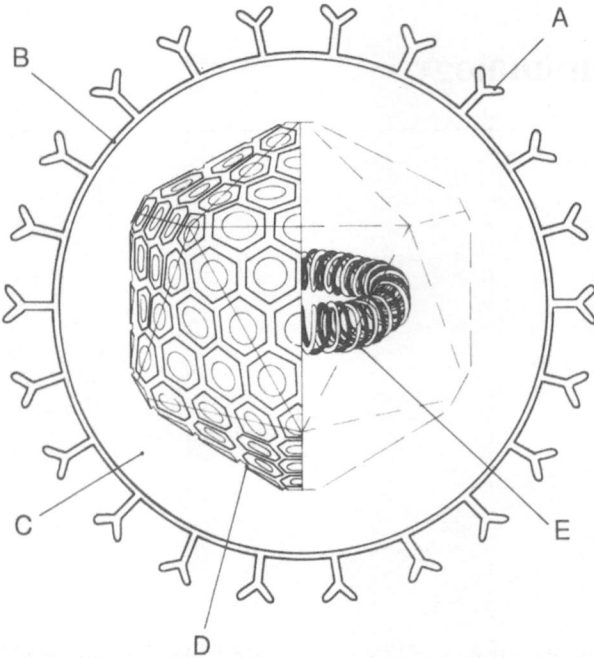

Fig. 1.1. Structure of herpes simplex virus.
A Viral glycoproteins: gB is required for infectivity, gC combines with C3b complement component, gD induces neutralising antibodies, gE binds to the FC portion of IgG, and gG is type specific for HSV 1 and for HSV 2. **B** Envelope. **C** Tegument containing specific proteins. **D** Capsid. **E** DNA.

Virology

Structure of HSV

The herpes virion consists of a DNA core, an iscosohedral capsid containing capsomers and an envelope. Between the capsid and the envelope is a structure, called the tegument, consisting of fibrous proteins. The diameter of the total enveloped virion measures 250 nm and that of the nucleocapsid approximately 100 nm (Fig. 1.1).

Envelope

The envelope is the outer covering of the virus, which is derived from modified host cell membranes as the DNA-containing capsid breaks through the nuclear membrane of the host cell (Roizman and Furlong 1974). It consists of a lipid bi-layer with five types of glycoprotein embedded in it. These glycoproteins mediate attachment of the virus to the host cell and are also important in allowing the virus to penetrate the cell membrane. Other functions include expression of Fc and complement receptors on the surface of infected cells, envelopment into the cytoplasm, and the egress and release of new virions. Glycoproteins are involved also in the spread of HSV from cell to cell (Spear 1984).

The glycoproteins identified so far are designated gB, gC, gD, gE and gG. Glycoproteins C and D appear to be the most important in binding the virus to the cell surface and gB is involved in penetration (Little et al. 1981). gC binds also to the C3b component of complement (Friedman et al. 1984) and gD is a potent inducer of neutralising antibodies. One of the roles of gE is to bind to the Fc portion of IgG (Bauke and Spear 1979). The functions of gG are yet to be determined. This glycoprotein is, however, type specific and antibodies to it have already been utilised in a type-specific serological assay (Lee et al. 1985, 1986; see also Chap. 7).

Capsid

The capsid consists of 162 capsomers arranged in an icosahedral symmetry. It is a highly rigid structure with 20 triangular facets and 12 corners (or apices). The laws of crystal structure determine the number of capsomers. Each apex consists of a single capsomer surrounded by five others (pentons). The non-apical capsomers are surrounded by six others (hexons). The virus therefore has 150 hexons and 12 pentons (Wildy et al. 1960). Other viruses with icosahedral symmetry have different numbers of capsomers (e.g. adenoviruses contain 252 capsomers and papovaviruses 72). The capsomers are made up of several types of polypeptide. They are shaped like hexagonal prisms with a hollow tube running the length of the long axis (Wildy et al. 1960).

Core

The core contains the viral DNA. The HSV genome is an extremely complex double-stranded linear DNA molecule with molecular weight 100×10^6 (Frenkel and Roizman 1971). HSV DNA consists of two covalently linked sequences, designated l (long) and s (short), comprising 82% and 18%, respectively, of the DNA. Each component consists of unique sequences Ul (unique long) and Us (unique short) bracketed by smaller inverted sequences. The two unique sequences can invert in relation to each other, so that the DNA extracted from HSV has been observed to occur in four different isomeric configurations, depending upon the relative orientation of the Ul and Us sequences (Roizman 1979).

Most of the genetic capacity of the virus is involved in coding for the large number of HSV polypeptides (probably well over 50). Three classes of polypeptide have been identified and designated α, β, and γ (the production and role of these proteins is discussed in detail below). However, the exact number and function of the genes and their products are yet to be determined.

The two HSVs have a considerable degree of genetic similarity, with approximately 50% of the sequences highly conserved. These sequences are found throughout the genomic map. In addition, many of the polypeptides specified by HSV 1 are antigenically related to those produced by HSV 2.

Viral Replication (Fig. 1.2)

In order for viral replication to occur, the genome needs to be transported through the cell surface and cytoplasm to the nucleus. This occurs as a result of three steps: (1) absorption of the virion into the cell surface, (2) penetration across the plasma membrane to the nuclear pore, and (3) uncoating of the capsid to release the viral DNA.

Absorption occurs when HSV attaches to the cell membrane, probably by means of one or more specific cell receptors. These receptors have not yet been identified. However, there is some evidence that HSV 1 and 2 each attach to different receptors (Vahlne et al. 1979, 1980). When the virus has attached to the cell surface, the viral envelope fuses with the cell membrane and the nucleocapsid is released into the cytoplasm (Morgan et al. 1968; DeLuca et al. 1981). Glycoprotein B may have a function in this process (Sarmiento et al. 1979). The nucleocapsid is transported to the nuclear pore, where the capsid is disassembled and the viral DNA released into the nucleus (Dales 1973).

Transcription of mRNAs occurs in the nucleus: HSV is believed not to have a virion transcriptase and viral RNA synthesis is probably catalysed by host cell RNA polymerase II. The mRNAs are then transported to the cytoplasm where translation into viral proteins occurs. The protein-synthesising capacity of the cell is slowly taken over. The majority of proteins produced are returned to the nucleus, which is also the site of DNA replication and reassembly of capsids.

Biosynthesis occurs in three phases in a highly regulated fashion (Honess and Roizman 1974). The mRNAs produced during each of these phases correspond to three grades of polypeptide α, β and γ; mRNA is translated during each of these phases fron non-contiguous areas of the viral DNA. Initially only α gene products are synthesised. They represent 10% of the genome and amongst their functions is the production of β proteins (Kozak and Roizman 1974; Honess and Roizman 1974). The β protein terminates α polypeptide production (in the cytoplasm) and starts the production of γ polypeptides (Fenwick and Roizman 1977; Honess and Roizman 1974). The β proteins include several regulatory proteins and enzymes (e.g. thymidine kinase and DNA polymerase) that are essential for DNA replication.

The final phase (the expression of γ genes and the production of γ proteins) follows the replication of viral DNA. The majority of the structural proteins of the virus are γ proteins. At the onset of viral DNA synthesis, β protein production ceases. In addition, host cellular DNA and protein syntheses are also terminated.

Assembly of viral capsids occurs in the nucleus when a critical concentration of viral structural proteins is reached. The capsids assume their icosahedral shape spontaneously (Vilček and Sreevalsan 1984).

Complete virions are probably transported to the cell membrane via the endoplasmic reticulum and the Golgi apparatus (Spear 1984). The glycosylation of the viral proteins that are inserted into the envelope probably also occurs in the Golgi apparatus. Possibly as a consequence of this, identical glycoproteins are found in the viral envelope and on the surface of infected cells. These glycoproteins carry specific antigenic determinants that may be important in the immune destruction of infected cells (Norrild et al. 1980).

It is presumed that the final release of complete infectious viral particles into the extracellular spaces and fluids occurs by a process of inverted endocytosis (Johnson and Spear 1982).

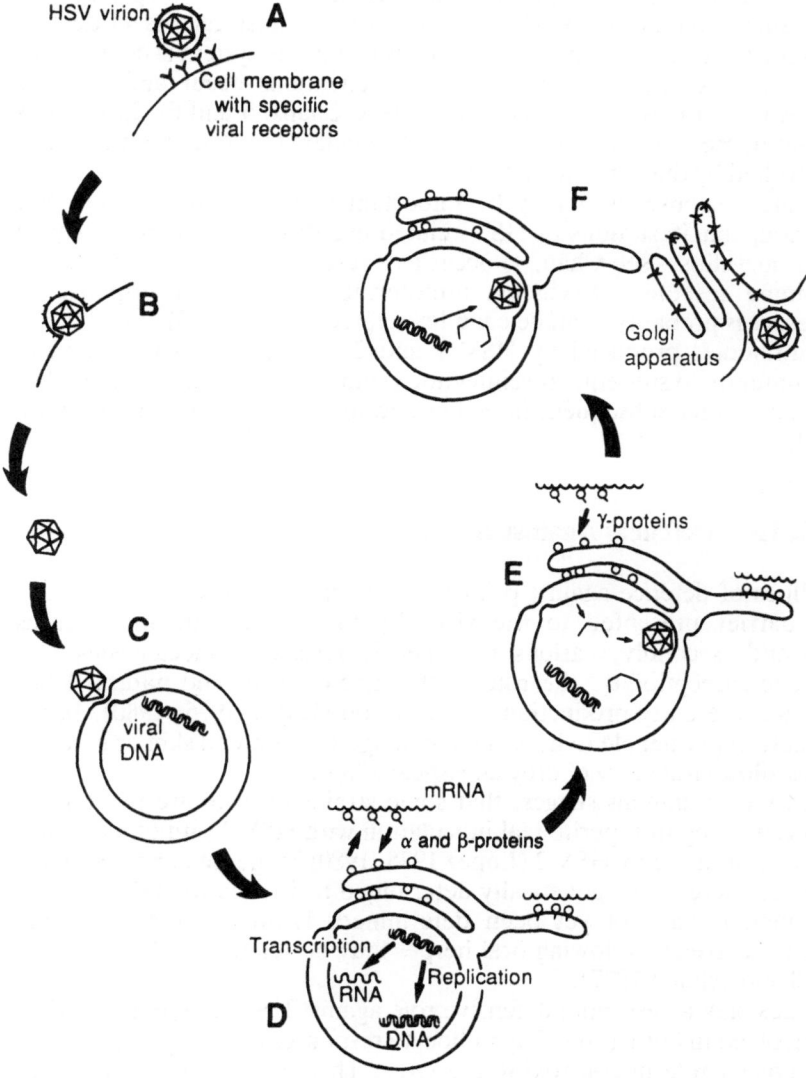

Fig. 1.2. Viral replication. **A** *HSV* attaches to a specific viral glycoprotein *receptors*. **B** Viral envelope merges with cell membrane and viral capsid enters the cytoplasm and is transported to the nucleus. **C** Disassembly of viral capsid and release of *viral DNA* into the nucleus. **D** Expression of α and β *proteins*. **E** Expression of γ *proteins*. Formation of new viral genome and capsid. Envelopment of virion as it "buds" through the inner nuclear membrane into the peri-nuclear space. **F** Transport to the *Golgi apparatus*, where glycosylation of viral proteins occurs. Release into the extracellular space.

Immunology

Introduction

A variety of immune responses both humoral and cellular occur as a result of infection with HSVs. These responses not only curtail the first episode and prevent dissemination of the virus but are also the host factors critical in maintaining the latent state of the virus. When the immune system is defective or damaged, latency is often not maintained, reactivations occur and in some circumstances the virus is able to disseminate (see Chaps. 5 and 6). In patients with recurrent herpes infections (oral, genital or ocular) the termination of each event is controlled by the immune system.

The immune response itself may be important in disease production. For example various manifestations of HSV-related eye disease (including stromal ulcers and iridocyclitis – see Chap. 4) occur as a result of tissue damage caused by the immune response. Erythema multiforme occurring in response to recurrent herpes is probably immune complex related (see Chap. 5).

Finally, antibodies produced by HSV 1 and 2, whilst not giving complete protective immunity to subsequent reinfection (with either the same or the other viral type), do modify subsequent infection and limit its severity and duration (see Chap. 4).

Non-specific Host Defences Against HSVs

The initial lines of defence against primary infection with herpes simplex are, firstly, the barrier presented to the virus by the intact skin and mucous membranes and, secondly, various non-specific resistance mechanisms that include genetic susceptibility, the role of the macrophages and natural killer (NK) cells, and the early production of interferon (Lopez 1975, 1980). Intact skin is probably impermeable to herpes but damaged or abraded skin or mucosal surfaces does allow viral entry (Corey and Spear 1986).

Experiments with animals suggest that some strains of mice are resistant to encephalitis caused by intraperitoneal inoculation with HSV 1 and other strains to focal hepatitis induced by HSV 2 (Lopez 1975, 1980; Mogensen and Andersen 1978). Whether there is any genetically determined resistance to HSV 1 and to HSV 2 in humans has not yet been determined. However, there is some evidence that recurrence following oral herpes may be related to HLA antigen type (Russell and Schlaut 1977).

Macrophages play an essential defensive role against HSV. Not only are they intimately involved in both T and B lymphocyte responses (discussed below) but they play a crucial role in controlling the virus. This involves phagocytosis of virions as well as retardation of viral replication by destroying virus-infected cells and by the release of interferon, which slows or stops the spread of virus to uninfected cells.

The exact function of NK cells in early protection against HSV is unknown. However, several observations support the view that NK cells are essential in early resistance to infection. NK cells exhibit non-specific cytotoxic activity against virus-infected or virally transformed cells. (Grewal et al. 1977; Herberman and Ortaldo 1981; Weigent et al. 1983; Welsh 1981). This cytotoxicity is enhanced by interferon (Gridlund et al. 1978; Zawatsky et al. 1981; Lopez et al. 1980). In patients with low NK cell counts, for example neonates and patients with Wiskott–Aldrich syndrome, severe, disseminated, life-threatening herpetic infections may occur (see Chaps. 5 and 6).

Finally, what is the role of interferons? HSV is a potent inducer of α interferon. Interferons increase the activity of various proteins and enzymes that may be involved in slowing or stopping viral replication (Rager-Zisman and Bloom 1974). However, the exact antiviral mechanisms and the relative importance of interferons in natural resistance to herpes viruses are still being investigated.

Antibody Production and Functions

In addition to the non-specific immunological mechanisms mentioned above, the host mounts both specific antibody and cell-mediated responses following infection with HSV.

Antibodies are produced to a host of viral proteins and glycoproteins (Zweerink and Stanton 1981; Zweerink and Corey 1982; Mann and Hilty 1982). The tests used to detect these antibodies and the various proteins and or glycoproteins detected are listed in Table 1.2. Antibodies to these various components appear to be produced sequentially (Zweerink and Stanton 1981; Eberle and Mou 1983; Ashley et al. 1985; Kahlon et al. 1986). The importance of each of the individual antibodies is unknown. However, a recent study of patients with genital herpes suggests that a lack of antibodies to three proteins (P66, g80 complex and gD) correlated with the early appearance of recurrences (Ashley et al. 1985). The majority of the antibodies to HSV 1 cross-react with HSV 2 and vice versa (Pereira et al. 1980; Norrild et al. 1980). However, antibodies directed towards glycoprotein G appear to be type specific and have been used to develop a type-specific serological assay (Lee et al. 1985, 1986).

In humans, the role of antibodies in containing the acute infection, in the development and maintenance of latency and in the relapse of infection is unclear. It is unlikely that antibodies are particularly important in limiting the extent of primary infections. Indeed, patients with defective humoral immunity

Table 1.2. Tests to detect HSV proteins and glycoproteins

Reactive proteins	Methods to detect	Immunoglobulin class
Membrane glycoproteins	Neutralisation	IgG/IgM
	Fluorescent microscopy	IgG/IgA/IgM
	Antibody-dependent immunocytologic tests	
	Complement mediated	IgG/IgM
	T cell mediated	IgG
Intracellular proteins	Neutralisation	IgG/IgM
Soluble infected-cell proteins	Immunoprecipitation	IgG
	Immunoblotting	IgG
Insoluble infected-cell proteins	Immunoblotting	IgG
Total or purified proteins	ELISA/RIA	IgG/IgA/IgM

ELISA, enzyme-linked immunosorbent assay; RIA, radio-immune assay.

do not develop more severe or prolonged primary infections than those with normal antibody production (Merigan and Stevens 1971).

Similar observations have been made in experimentally infected mice, where local skin infections are no more severe in B cell-suppressed mice than in those with normal immunity (Kapoor et al. 1982; Simmons and Nash 1984). However, antibody to HSV has been shown to limit the extent of spread within the peripheral nervous system thereby possibly limiting the extent of latently infected neurones (Simmons and Nash 1987).

In contrast to the situation with primary infection, in recurrent disease and with reinfection antibodies appear to be very important. Patients with recurrent herpetic infections usually have high levels of neutralising HSV antibody (Nahmias and Roizman 1973). These antibodies may be important in limiting the extent of each recurrence, probably by assisting the destruction of virus-infected cells by complement and/or NK cells (Jayasuriya and Nash 1985), as well as by acting synergistically with unsensitised cells to lyse the infected cells. This process is called antibody-dependent cell-mediated cytotoxicity (Shore et al. 1976). The Fc portion of anti-HSV antibodies is apparently important for the process (Hayashida et al. 1982).

Antibodies also have an effect when the individual is exposed to HSV of one or other viral type. Indeed patients with previous exposure to HSV 1, usually at the oral site, have a less severe infection when subsequently exposed to HSV 2 at the genital site (Corey et al. 1983), and it is possible that some will not develop any clinical illness.

It is evident from animal experiments that passively acquired antibody (to known viral glycoproteins B, C, D, E and G) may offer protection against subsequent challenge with virulent virus (Chan 1983; Dix and Mills 1985; Meignier et al. 1987; Balachandran et al. 1982). These experiments form the theoretical basis for the production of some HSV vaccines and are discussed in more detail in Chap. 8.

The same does not appear to be true in humans, where passively transferred maternal antibodies do not appear to prevent neonates from developing herpes (Whitley et al. 1980). Although antibodies may modify the severity of the illness (Nahmias et al. 1983; see also Chap. 5). Although we now know that antibodies are produced to a vast array of HSV proteins and glycoproteins, it is unknown whether any one of these is more important than any other in terms of protection. Nor do we know whether the presence of any one antibody or combination of antibodies confers or indeed can predict protection from recurrences or subsequent reinfection (Corey and Spear 1986).

Cell-mediated Immunity

Unlike the situation with antibody-mediated immunity, cell-mediated immunity (CMI) is essential for recovery from herpes during both the first attack and subsequent relapses. Patients with depressed CMI, for example those with malignancy, severe infection or AIDS, often have severe mucocutaneous or disseminated herpetic infections (see Chap. 5).

T cells appear to play a primary role in controlling herpes. The evidence for this comes largely from animal experiments, but there is some evidence from studies in humans. Firstly, as mentioned above, patients with depressed CMI (and therefore decreased or malfunctioning T cells) are prone to severe herpetic infection (Muller et al. 1972; Graham and Snell 1983; Siegal et al. 1981). An example of this is infection due to the human immunodeficiency virus (HIV), where the prime immunological deficit is the destruction of T helper/inducer cells by the virus; patients are particularly prone to severe and progressive HSV infections (Siegal et al. 1981; Midlvan et al. 1982; Clumek et al. 1984). Secondly, studies in patients with oral herpes have shown that virus-specific T cell subsets are activated during recurrences (Tsutsumi et al. 1986) and Corey et al. (1979) were able to show that the cellular immune response was important in patients with genital herpes.

In contrast to the limited information from humans, there is an enormous literature relating to cellular immunity in animals experimentally infected with HSV. The importance of thymus-derived lymphocytes in protection against HSV infection has been demonstrated in numerous studies. Neonatally thymectomised mice and those with congenital thymic defects (athymic nude mice) have been shown to be highly susceptible to progressive HSV infection (Mori et al. 1967; Kapoor et al. 1982; Nagafuchi et al. 1979). Similar susceptibility to progressive HSV infection has been demonstrated in other forms of immunosuppression, including exposure to X-irradiation, treatment with cyclophosphamide and infection with anti-thymocyte serum (Oakes 1975; Rager-Zisman and Allison 1976). In neonatally thymectomised mice, the infection can be controlled by subsequently injecting the mice with immune T cells (Kapoor et al. 1982).

Delayed-Type Hypersensitivity and T Cell Responses

There is still considerable debate as to which T cells mediate protection, and there is evidence suggesting that T cells involved in both cytotoxicity and delayed-type hypersensitivity (DTH) may be important.

Subcutaneous injection of HSV into mouse ear has proved to be an excellent model for investigating DTH responses (Nash et al. 1980a, 1981a). The DTH response depends on the recruitment of effector cells, including macrophage and monocytes, to the site of infection. This cellular recruitment is mediated by lymphokines released by antigen-activated T cells of the DTH group.

HSV-specific T DTH cells can be recovered from the draining lymph nodes 4–10 days after inoculation. Subsequent injection of these cells into non-immune mice has been shown to confer both DTH and antiviral immunity. The appearance of T DTH cells correlates with the time when virus is rapidly eliminated from mouse ear pinna (Greene and Weiner 1980). Protection by DTH cells is considered to be mediated by cells restricted by the major histocompatibility complex (MHC) class II markers (Nash et al. 1981b).

Cytotoxic T Cell Responses

In contrast to DTH responses, which are mediated by MHC class II restricted cells, the cytotoxic responses are mediated by MHC class I.

Using the mouse ear model mentioned above, it has been shown that cytotoxic T lymphocytes (CTLs) can be detected in the draining lymph nodes 4 days after inoculation, reaching a peak by 6–9 days (Nash et al. 1980b). CTLs recognise both type-common and type-specific HSV antigens (Eberle et al. 1981; Carter et al. 1982). HSV-primed CTLs can apparently transfer resistance to non-infected mice (Larson et al. 1983) and more recent work with a cloned CTL line specific for HSV has been shown to have a similar protective effect (Sethi et al. 1983).

In the mouse model it is apparent that both DTH and cytotoxic T cells are important in controlling the spread of acute HSV infections.

T Suppressor Cells

The importance of T suppressor cells in the control of the acute infection and in the pathogenesis of recurrences is unknown. It has been suggested that T suppressor cells may suppress DTH and thus be important in the production of recurrences (Jayasuriya and Nash 1985), but the experimental evidence supporting this is scanty (Nash et al. 1981c; Schrier et al. 1983).

Role of the Immune System in Latency and Reactivation

The immune system may play an important part in the production and maintenance of latency and in subsequent viral reactivation. The mechanisms involved and the evidence supporting this view are discussed in Chap. 2.

Conclusions

There is now considerable evidence from experimentally infected mice that both humoral immunity and cellular immunity are important in controlling HSV infections, together with the non-specific host defence mechanisms.

In primary infections, NK cells and interferons are probably vital in the early control of HSV infections. Subsequent activation of T cells including both DTH T cells and cytotoxic T cells would appear to be important in the elimination of the first attack, and in preventing its dissemination and spread. As antibodies are produced only late in the infection, their role in controlling the primary infection is probably limited.

Antibodies appear to play a vital part in limiting the extent of each recurrence by assisting the destruction of cells infected with virus by complement or NK cells, as well as through the process of antibody-dependent cell-mediated cytotoxicity.

What is the role of the immune system in controlling HSV infections in humans? Both humoral immunity and cellular immunity appear to be important. However, very few detailed studies have been done. It is well known that patients with depressed CMI can develop severe disseminated HSV infections, but studies of CMI in immunocompetent patients are few and far between. Recent interest in the immune responses (both cellular and humoral) to specific epitopes of viral polypeptides and glycoproteins, coupled with more sophisticated techniques for studying these responses, will it is hoped lead to a better understanding of these mechanisms in the coming years.

References

Ashley R, Benedetti J, and Corey L (1985) Humoral immune response to HSV 1 and HSV 2 viral proteins in patients with primary genital herpes. J Med Virol 17: 153–166

Balachandran N, Bacchetti S, Rawls WE (1982) Protection against lethal challenge of BALB/c mice by passive transfer of monoclonal antibodies to five glycoproteins of herpes simplex virus type 2. Infect Immun 37: 1132–1137

Bauke RB, Spear PG (1979) Membrane proteins specified by herpes simplex viruses. V. Identification of an Fc-binding glycoprotein. J Virol 46: 103–112

Carter VC, Rice PL, Tevethia SS (1982) Intratypic and intertypic specificity of lymphocytes involved in recognition of herpes simplex virus glycoproteins. Infect Immun 37: 116–126

Chan WL (1983) Protective immunization of mice with specific HSV 1 glycoproteins. Immunology 49: 343–352

Clumek N, Sonnet J, Taelman H (1984) Acquired immunodeficiency syndrome in African patients. N Engl J Med 310: 492–497

Corey L, Spear PG (1986) Infection with herpes simplex viruses. (first of two parts.) N Engl J Med 314:686–691

Corey L, Reeves WC, Holmes KK (1979) Cellular immune response in genital herpes simplex virus infection. N Engl J Med 299: 986–991

Corey L, Adams HG, Brown ZA, Holmes KK (1983) Genital herpes simplex virus infections. Clinical manifestations, course and complications. Ann Intern Med 98: 958–972

Dales S (1973) Early events in cell–animal virus interactions. Bacteriol Rev 37: 103–135

DeLuca N, Bzik D, Person S, Snipes W (1981) Early events in herpes simplex virus type 1 infection; photosensitivity of fluorescein isothiocyanate-treated virions. Proc Natl Acad Sci USA 78: 912–916

Dix RD, Mills J (1985) Acute and latent herpes simplex viruses. Neurological diseases in mice immunized with purified glycoproteins gB or gD. J Med Virol 17: 9–18

Eberle R, Mou SW (1983) Relative titres of antibodies to individual polypeptide antigens of herpes simplex virus type 1 human sera. J Infect Dis 148: 443–444

Eberle R, Russell RG, Rouse BT (1981) Cell mediated immunity to herpes simplex virus: recognition of type-specific and type-common surface antigens by cytotoxic T cell populations. Infect Immun 34: 795–803

Fenwick M, Roizman B (1977) Regulation of herpesvirus macromolecular synthesis. VI Synthesis and modification of viral polypeptides in enucleated cells. J Virol 22: 720–725

Frenkel N, Roizman B (1971) Herpes simplex virus: genome size and redundancy studied by renaturation kinetics. J Virol 8: 591–593

Friedman HM, Cohen GH, Eisenberg RJ, Seidel CA, Cines DB (1984) Glycoproteins C of herpes simplex virus 1 as a receptor for the C3b complement component on infected cells. Nature 309: 633–635

Graham BS, Snell JD (1983) Herpes simplex virus infection of the adult lower respiratory tract. Medicine (Baltimore) 62: 384–393

Greene MI, Weiner HL (1980) Delayed hypersensitivity in mice infected with reovirus. II. Induction of tolerance and suppressor T cells to viral specific gene products. J Immunol 125: 283–287

Grewal AS, Rouse BT, Babiuk LA (1977) Mechanisms of resistance to herpesvirus: comparison of the effectiveness of different cell types in mediating antibody-dependent cell-mediated cytoxicity. Infect Immun 15: 698–703

Gridlund M, Orn A, Wigzell H, Senik A, Gresser I (1978) Enhanced NK cell activity in mice infected with interferon and interferon inducers. Nature 273: 759–761

Hayashida I, Nagafuchi S, Hayashi Y et al (1982) Mechanism of antibody-mediated protection against herpes simplex virus infection in athymic mice: requirement of Fc portion of antibody. Microbiol Immunol 26: 497–509

Herberman RB, Ortaldo JR (1981) Natural killer cells. Their role in defenses against disease. Science 214: 24–30

Honess RW, Roizman B (1974) Regulation of herpesvirus macromolecular synthesis in cascade regulation of the synthesis of 3 groups of viral proteins. J Virol 14: 8–19

Jayasuriya AK, Nash AA (1985) Pathogenesis and immunobiology of herpes simplex virus in mouse and man. Cancer Invest 3: 199–207

Johnson DC, Spear PG (1982) Monensin inhibits the processing of herpes simplex virus glycoproteins, their transport to the cell surface and the egress of virions from infected cells. J Virol 43: 1102–1112

Kahlon J, Lakeman FD, Ackermann M, Whitley RJ (1986) Human antibody response to herpes simplex virus specific polypeptides after primary and recurrent infection. J Clin Microbiol 23: 725–730

Kapoor AK, Nash AA, Wildy P (1982) Pathogenesis of herpes simplex virus in B cell-suppressed mice: the relative roles of cell mediated and humoral immunity. J Gen Virol 61: 127–131

Kozak M, Roizman B (1974) Regulation of herpesvirus macromolecular synthesis: nuclear retention of non-translated viral RNA sequences. Proc Natl Acad Sci USA 71: 4322-4326

Larson HS, Russel RG, Rouse BT (1983) Recovery from lethal herpes simplex virus type 1 infection is mediated by cytotoxic T lymphocyte. Infect Immun 41: 197–204

Lee FK, Coleman RM, Pereira L, Bailey PD, Tatsuno M, Nahmias AJ (1985) Detection of herpes simplex virus type 2 specific antibody with glycoprotein G. J Clin Microbiol 22: 641–644

Lee FK, Pereira L, Griffin C, Reid E, Nahmias A (1986) A novel glycoprotein for detection of herpes simplex virus type 1 specific antibodies. Virol Methods 14: 111–118

Little SP, Jofre JT, Courtney RJ, Schaffer PA (1981) A virion-associated glycoprotein essential for infectivity of herpes simplex virus type 1. Virology 115: 149–160

Lopez C (1975) Genetics of natural resistance to herpes virus infections in mice. Nature 258: 152–153

Lopez C (1980) Genetic resistance to herpes infection. Role of natural killer cells. In: Skamene E, Kongshaun P, Landy M (eds) Genetic control of natural resistance to infection and malignancy. Acadamic Press, New York, pp 253–265

Mann D, Hilty M (1982) Antibody response to herpes simplex virus type 1 polypeptides and glycoproteins in primary and recurrent infection. Pediatr Res 16: 176–186

Meignier B, Jourdier TM, Norrild B, Pereira L, Roizman B (1987) Immunization of experimental animals with reconstituted glycoprotein mixtures of herpes simplex virus 1 and 2. Protection against challenge with virulent virus. J Infect Dis 155: 921–930

Merigan TC, Stevens DA (1971) Viral infection in man associated with acquired immunological deficiency states. Fed Proc 30: 1858–1864

Midlvan D, Mathur U, Enslow RW, et al (1982) Opportunistic infections and immune deficiency in homosexual men. Ann Intern Med 69: 700-704

Mogensen SC, Andersen HK (1978) Role of activated macrophages in resistance of congenitally athymic nude mice to hepatitis induced by herpes simplex type 2. Infect Immun 19: 792–798

Morgan C, Rose HM, Mednis B (1968) Electron microscopy of herpes simplex virus. I. Entry. J Virol 2: 507–516

Mori R, Tasaki T, Kimura G, Takeya K (1967) Depression of acquired resistance against herpes simplex virus infection in neonatally thymectomized mice. Arch Ges Virusforsch 21: 459–462

Muller SA, Herrman EC, Winkelmann RK (1972) Herpes simplex infections in hematologic malignancies. Am J Med 52: 102–114

Nagafuchi S, Oda H, Mori R, Taniguchi T (1979) Mechanism of acquired resistance to herpes simplex virus infection as studied in nude mice. J Gen Virol 44: 715–723

Nahmias AJ, Roizman B (1973) Infection with herpes simplex viruses 1 and 2. (First of three parts.) N Engl J Med 667–674

Nahmias AJ, Keyserling HH, Kerrick G (1983) Herpes simplex. In: Remington JS, Klein JO (eds) Infectious diseases of the fetus and newborn infant. WB Saunders, Philadelphia, PA, pp 156–190

Nash AA, Field HJ, Quartey-Papafio R (1980a) Cell mediated immunity to herpes simplex virus-infected mice: induction, characterisation and antiviral effects of delayed-type hypersensitivity. J Gen Virol 48: 351–357

Nash AA, Quartey-Papafio R, Wildy P (1980b) Cell-mediated immunity in herpes simplex virus-infected mice: functional analysis of lymph nodes cells during periods of acute and latent infection, with reference to cytotoxic and memory cells. J Gen Virol 49: 309–317

Nash AA, Gell PGH, Wildy P (1981a) Tolerance and immunity in mice infected with herpes simplex virus: simultaneous induction of protective immunity and tolerance to delayed-type hypersensitivity. Immunology 43: 153–159

Nash AA, Phelan J, Wildy P (1981b) Cell-mediated immunity in herpes simplex virus infected mice: H2-mapping of the delayed-type hypersensitivity response and the antiviral T cell response. J Immunol 126: 1260–1262

Nash AA, Phelan J,. Gell PGH, Wildy P (1981c) Tolerance and immunity in mice infected with herpes simplex virus: studies on the mechanism of tolerance to delayed-type hypersensitivity. Immunology 43: 363–364

Norrild B, Shore SL, Cromeans TL, Nahmias AJ (1980) Participation of three major glycoprotein antigens of herpes simplex virus type 1 early in the infectious cycle as determined by antibody dependent cell-mediated cytotoxicity. Infect Immun 28: 38–44

Oakes JE (1975) Role for cell mediated immunity in the resistance of mice to subcutaneous herpes simplex infection. Infect Immunol 12: 166–172

Pereira L, Klassen T, Baringer J (1980) Type common and type specific monoclonal antibodies to herpes simplex virus type 1. Infect Immun 29: 724-732

Rager-Zisman B, Bloom BR (1974) Immunological destruction of herpes simplex virus 1 infected cells. Nature 251: 542–543

Rager-Zisman B, Allison AC (1976) Mechanisms of immunologic resistance to herpes simplex virus (HSV 1) infection. J Immunol 116: 35–40

Roizman B (1979) The organisation of the herpes simplex virus genomes. Annu Rev Genet 13: 25–57

Roizman B, Furlong D (1974) The replication of herpesviruses. In: Fraekel-Conrat H, Wagner RR (eds) Comprehensive virology, Plenum Press, New York pp 229–403

Russell AS, Schlaut J (1977) Association of HLA-A1 antigen and susceptibility to recurrent cold sores. Arch Dermatol 113: 1721–1722

Sarmiento M, Haffey M, Spear PG (1979) Membrane proteins specified by herpes simplex viruses. III. Role of glycoproteins VP7 (B2) in virion infectivity. J Virol 29: 1149–1158

Schrier RD, Pizer LI, Moorhead JW (1983) Tolerance and suppression of immunity to herpes simplex virus; different presentation of antigen induced different types of suppressor cells. Infect Immun 40: 514–522

Sethi KK, Omata Y, Schneweis KE (1983) Protection of mice from fatal herpes simplex virus type 1 infection by adoptive transfer of cloned virus-specified and H 2 restricted cytotoxic T lymphocytes. J Gen Virol 64: 443–447

Shore SL, Cromeans TL, Romano TJ (1976) Immune destruction of virus infected cells early in the infectious cycle. Nature 262: 695–696

Siegal FP, Lopez C, Hammer GS, et al. (1981) Severe acquired immunodeficiency in male homosexuals, manifested by chronic perianal ulcerative herpes simplex lesions. N Engl J Med 305: 1439–1444

Simmons A, Nash AA (1984) Zosteriform species of herpes simplex virus as a model of recrudescence and its use to investigate the roll of immune cells in prevention of recurrent disease. J Virol 52: 816–821

Simmons A, Nash AA (1987) Effect of B cell suppression on primary infection and reinfection of mice with herpes simplex virus. J Infect Dis 155: 649–654

Spear PG (1984) Glycoproteins specified by herpes simplex virus. In: Roizmann B. (ed) The herpesviruses, vol 3, Plenum Press, New York, pp 315–356

Tsutsumi H, Bernstein JM, Riepenhoff-Talty M, Cohen E, Orsini F, Ogra PL (1986) Immune responses to herpes simplex virus in patients with recurrent herpes labialis. I. Development of cell mediated cytotoxic responses. Clin Exp Immunol 66: 507–515

Vahlne A, Svennerholm B, Lycke E (1979) Evidence for herpes simplex virus type-selective receptors on cellular plasma membranes. J Gen Virol 44: 217–225

Vahlne A, Svennerholm B, Sandberg M, Hamberger A, Lycke E (1980) Differences in attachment between herpes simplex virus type 1 and type 2 viruses to neurones and glial cells. Infect Immun 28: 675–680

Vilček J, Sreevalsan T (1984) Fundamentals of virus structure and replication. In: Galasso G J, Merrigan TC, Buchanan RA (eds) Antiviral agents and viral diseases of man, 2nd edn, Raven Press, New York, pp 1–33

Weigent DA, Langford MP, Fleischmann WR Jr, Stanton GJ (1983) Potentiation of lymphocyte natural killing by mixture of alpha or beta interferon with recombinant gamma interferon. Infect Immun 40: 35–38

Welsh RM (1981) Natural cell-mediated immunity during viral infection. Curr Top Microbiol Immunol 92: 83–106

Whitley RJ, Nahmias AJ, Visintine AM, Fleming CL, Alford CA (1980) The natural history of herpes simplex virus of mother and newborn. Pediatrics 66: 489–494

Wildy P, Russell WC, Horne RW (1960) The morphology of herpes virus. Virology 12: 1044–1052

Zawatsky R, Hilfenhaus J, Marcucci F, Kirchner H (1981) Experimental infection of inbred mice with herpes simplex type 1. I. Investigation of humoral and cellular immunity of interferon induction. J Gen Virol 53: 31–38

Zweerink H, Corey L (1982) Virus-specific antibodies in sera from patients with genital herpes simplex virus infection. Infect Immun 37: 413–421

Zweerink H, Stanton L (1981) Immune response to herpes simplex virus infections: virus specific antibodies in sera from patients with recurrent facial infections. Infect Immun 31: 624–630

Chapter 2

Latency and Oncogenesis

Latency

Introduction

Most human herpes viruses (HSV types 1 and 2, varicella zoster (VZV), cytomegalovirus (CMV) and the Epstein–Barr virus (EBV)) are able to establish latency. Whether the recently described human herpes virus–6 (HHV–6; Tedder et al. 1987) can do so is yet to be determined. Clinical reactivations of CMV, EBV and VZV occur rarely, but such reactivations occur commonly with HSV, even in individuals with normal immunity. The concept that repeated episodes of HSV occurred as a result of reactivation rather than reinfection arose from several observations: both oral and genital HSV often recur at the same anatomical site; certain physical and emotional events could precipitate recurrences; and serum HSV antibody levels are relatively consistent irrespective of how often lesions occur (Hill et al. 1984).

Although the concept of latency was first postulated 60 years ago (Goodpasture 1929), it is only in the last 20 years, with the ability to culture HSV, the development of animal models, and recent advances in molecular biology, that mechanisms of latency and reactivation have begun to be understood. However, our understanding of this complex issue is far from complete and numerous questions and controversies remain.

Establishment of Latency

Acute Phase

HSV enters the host through mucocutaneous surfaces. What happens next is the subject of some controversy. It was originally believed that the virus replicated at the inoculation site (giving rise to the typical herpetic lesions), was then taken up by sensory nerve terminals with special viral receptors (Vahlne et al. 1978), penetrated the nerve axon as part of the replication process (Lycke et al. 1984), and was finally translocated centripetally by retrograde axonal spread (Kristensson 1978). Animal experiments suggest that these events may be more complex. Using a mouse model, inoculated virus was shown to reach a peak titre 2 days after inoculation at the site of the original infection, but could not be found in surrounding skin. Over the following 2–3 days, virus was found in the surrounding tissue, eventually forming typical herpetic lesions over the entire dermatome. Severing of the nerves serving that dermatone prevented the development of typical herpetic lesions (Simmons and Nash 1984; Blyth et al. 1984). These experiments suggest that there is an early and rapid movement of virus up and down the nerves, that latency is established very early and that HSV may be immunologically privileged soon after the initial exposure (Wildy 1985). These findings are of considerable practical importance, as they suggest that latency is unlikely to be prevented with antiviral therapy unless such therapy is initiated within 48 h of exposure.

Replication of HSV in Neurones

HSV replication is usually associated with cell death, but this does not appear to be the case with neurones. Several possible explanations have been offered. The first is that viral replication may not be necessary for the establishment of latency. This view is supported by experiments using temperature-sensitive (ts) mutants of HSV 1. These experiments showed that ts mutants that did not replicate at non-permissive body temperature were still capable of inducing latency in mice (Lofgren et al. 1977; Watson et al. 1980).

Openshaw et al (1981) offered two additional alternative explanations. Firstly, they suggested that sensory ganglia may contain two types of neurones. Permissive neurones would allow for establishment of latency, whilst non-permissive ones would act as reservoirs for both retrograde and antegrade dissemination. A second suggestion is that all ganglion cells are permissive for HSV, but that the subsequent immune response modulates productive infection, limiting it to a non-lytic latent infection. This would be similar to the immune response in measles (Joseph and Oldstone 1974).

Animal experiments have shown that HSV-encoded thymidine kinase (TK) is required for the establishment of latency (Tenser et al. 1979, 1981; Becker et al. 1984; Field and Darby 1980; Price and Khan 1981). Price (1985) has offered three possible explanations for this. Firstly, TK may be required for amplification of replication of the inoculum within the epithelium, thereby producing sufficient viral titres to ensure the seeding of nerve terminals. Secondly, TK itself may be necessary to initiate, establish or maintain latency. The final explanation is that TK-deficient virus may establish latency, but may be unable to reactivate. Viral gene products other than TK may also be important in regulating viral gene expression and modulating host cell expression (Price 1985; Lofgren et al. 1977; Watson et al. 1980).

Maintenance of Latency

Once latency is established, there exists an unstable relationship between the viral gene and the host neuronal cells. The exact nature of this relationship is largely unknown, as are the exact cellular and/or virological events leading to reactivation.

State of the Virus

The fundamental question with regard to the maintenance of latency is "what is the molecular state of the virus during this phase?" It is unknown whether or not HSV DNA is in an episomal form – either linear as it exists naturally in virions or circularised through terminal replications (Cantin et al. 1984) – or is integrated into host cellular DNA. It is possible that both episomal and integrated forms exist as with EBV (Lindahl et al. 1976). There is evidence to support each of these possibilities. The detection of terminal genomic fragments of a molecular size identical with that of virion DNA in the brains of experimentally infected mice suggests that these fragments are part of free linear DNA molecules (Kastoukoff et al. 1981). Rock and Fraser (1983) using Southern blot hybridisation suggested that the detection of genomic fragments in the brains of acutely infected mice (but not in those with latent infection) was evidence that the HSV genome was present in a form other than linear – possibly a circular or concatameric structure. Replicative intermediates that accumulate when HSV is grown in tissue culture are believed to be similar. Finally, experiments using restriction enzyme analysis with biopsies from the trigeminal ganglia of latently infected mice points to the possibility either that the HSV genome may be integrated into cellular DNA or that the molecular structure has been rearranged (Puga et al. 1984). How applicable are these studies in relation to latency in humans remains unknown.

What about gene transcription during latency? Experiments by Puga et al. (1978) using reassociation hybridisation kinetics showed that HSV DNA was detectable at a level of O.1 genome equivalents per ganglion cell of latently infected mice, but mRNA was not detected. In seeming contrast, Galloway and her team (1979) were able to detect HSV mRNA in up to 8% of the neurones from sensory ganglia derived from the sacral, thoracic and lumbar regions of humans. Subsequent experiments using cloned DNA genomic fragments showed hybridisation with a fragment of the genome which included the TK gene (Galloway et al. 1982). These experiments suggest that some transcription is occurring during latency. There is some other experimental evidence to support this view, including studies in experimentally infected mice showing detection of HSV 1 TK in the root ganglia up to 60 days after inoculation (Yamamoto et al. 1977) and detection of the immediate early viral polypeptide VP175 in trigeminal ganglia of infected rabbits (Green et al. 1981).

Recent studies using hybridisation in situ from the neurones both of experimentally infected mice (Stevens et al. 1987) and of humans (Croen et al. 1987) suggest that an RNA species complementary to that encoding an early gene transcript can be detected during latency. In contrast, the normal (also called "sense") transcript can be found during active viral replication. It is possible that this complementary ("anti-sense") transcript may be important in maintaining latency by blocking the production of immediate early genes and consequently the active production of infection.

Special Features of Neurones

Doerfler (1981) showed that gene expression in eukaryotic cells was linked to the methylation of cytosine residues in DNA. Expression of genes require little or no methylation, whereas silent genes are heavily methylated. Because of the high degree of differentiation and therefore limited gene expression in neurones, neuronal DNA is likely to be highly methylated.

HSV DNA gene expression may also be regulated by methylation (Hill et al. 1984; Youssoufian et al. 1982). The likelihood that neuronal DNA is highly methylated and the observation that HSV DNA gene expression may be dependent on the level of such methylation suggest that neurones are ideal cells for the establishment of HSV latency. The degree of DNA methylation may be important in both the maintenance of latency and subsequent viral reactivation (see below).

Summary and Conclusion (Fig. 2.1)

The above evidence suggests that the virus is unlikely to be totally inactive during latency (the so-called "static theory"): rather low levels of gene expression probably occur (the "dynamic theory"). Numerous factors may be important in maintaining the balance between low-level gene expression and active viral replication. These include the number of neurones infected, the degree of methylation in neuronal DNA, the role of the immune system during latency, and extraneous host factors such as trauma, infection and menstruation.

Viral Reactivation

Introduction

Several events are thought to be associated with recurrences of herpes. These may be divided into host factors and viral factors. Let us consider host factors first. With orolabial herpes, these may include exposure to cold, sunlight and wind, dental procedures, infectious diseases, emotional stress, fatigue and menstruation (Overall 1984; Spruance et al. 1977); with genital herpes, the factors are sexual intercourse, stress, fatigue and menstruation (Reeves et al. 1981; Guinan et al. 1981; Mindel et al. 1988). Immune suppression, particularly in relation to tumours, chemotherapy and infection with the human immunodeficiency virus (HIV), may also be important in the development of recurrences (see Chaps. 1 and 5). In experimental animals a variety of stimuli can cause reactivation; these include nerve section, treatment with cyclophosphamide and 6-hydroxydopamine, X-rays, application of dry ice, and superinfection with pneumococci (Hill 1984; Price 1979).

What about viral factors? It is possible that both viral type and "strain" variation may be important in determining the likelihood and frequency of recurrences. Several studies have shown that genital infections with HSV 2 are more likely to recur, and to recur with greater frequency, than those due to HSV 1 (Reeves et al. 1981; Mindel and Sutherland 1983). However, a recent study by

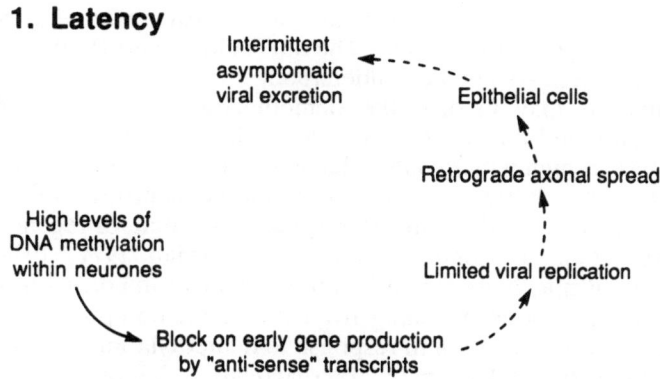

1. Latency

Intermittent asymptomatic viral excretion

Epithelial cells

Retrograde axonal spread

High levels of DNA methylation within neurones

Limited viral replication

Block on early gene production by "anti-sense" transcripts

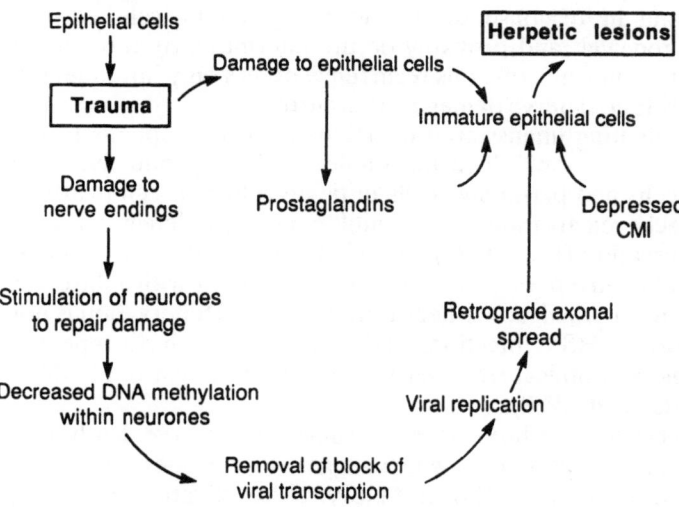

2. Reactivation

Epithelial cells

Trauma

Damage to epithelial cells

Herpetic lesions

Immature epithelial cells

Damage to nerve endings

Prostaglandins

Depressed CMI

Stimulation of neurones to repair damage

Retrograde axonal spread

Decreased DNA methylation within neurones

Viral replication

Removal of block of viral transcription

Fig. 2.1. Pathogenesis of HSV *latency* and *reactivation*. *CMI*, cell-mediated immunity.

Lafferty et al. (1987) suggests that recurrences may be due not only to the viral type but also to the site involved. Whilst they were able to confirm previous observations that HSV 2 recurred more frequently at the genital site than did HSV 1, they also showed that HSV 1 recurred more frequently at the oral site than did HSV 2.

What of strain variation? It has been postulated that different strains of HSV 1 or 2 may differ in their ability to reactivate (Sutherland et al. 1986). To date there is no convincing evidence to support this hypothesis.

Mechanism

The majority of "stimuli" resulting in viral reactivation probably involve some degree of nerve damage and it has been suggested that the anabolic neuronal response to injury may be the trigger that switches limited (or no) viral gene expression to synthesis of progeny (Price 1985). The molecular events (both host and viral) involved in this switch are not well understood.

One possible mechanism may involve the demethylation of host DNA (Doerfler 1981). As mentioned above, neurones normally have limited gene expression and their DNA is highly methylated. However, in response to injury (albeit minor) the cell responds by switching from routine neurotransmitter maintenance to the production of cellular macromolecules essential for regeneration of the damaged axons or nerve terminals (Lieberman 1971, 1974; Kreutzberg 1982). The virus may have adapted to these changes in normal host metabolism, with its own functions switching from low-level, non-productive gene expression to active viral replication in response to demethylation of DNA within the host cell. If this is the mechanism of viral reactivation, it is presumably terminated when the host response ceases.

The fact that the virus may be isolated from mucosal surfaces in the absence of symptoms or typical herpetic lesions (see Chaps. 3 and 4) suggests that reactivation is occurring in response to the normal physiological neuronal process of repair and renewal, and probably occurs intermittently throughout the life of the individual. Clinically obvious recurrence occurs only infrequently, perhaps when more substantial nerve damage has occurred.

One of the most fascinating unanswered questions is "what happens to the neurone during viral reactivation?" The inevitable result of productive viral infection in epithelial cells and permissive cells in tissue culture is cell death. If neurones die with each reactivation one would expect to detect an ever increasing area of denervation (Price 1985), especially in patients with frequent clinical recurrences, and recurrences would either cease or occur with a different dermatomal distribution. In practice, neither of these occurs. Denervation is not a consequence of recurrent HSV infections and many patients have repeated recurrences at the same anatomical site over many years (Guinan et al. 1981; Corey et al. 1983; Mindel et al. 1988).

Despite clinical observations on humans which suggest that nerve death does not occur, there are animal experiments which suggest that it does. Studies in experimentally infected mice have shown that viral reactivation following neurectomy or the use of 6-hydroxydopamine during the acute phase resulted in a decrease in latency (Price 1979; Price and Schmitz 1979). Using immunofluorescence to detect latent foci in cultures of explanted ganglia from experimentally infected mice, McLennan and Darby (1980) showed that repeated reactivation resulted in a decrease in the number of foci. All of these findings are in keeping with cell death occurring with recurrences. Finally, electron micrographs of the trigeminal ganglia of latently infected mice showed abnormal neurones surrounded by macrophages – perhaps reflecting cell death from spontaneous viral reactivation (Baringer and Swoveland 1974). It is likely that the pathogenesis of latency in experimental animals is very different from that occurring naturally in humans. If, as seems likely from clinical observation, neuronal death does not occur, we are left with the intriguing and as yet unanswered problem of how viral replication occurs without irretrievable host cell damage.

Viral Transport and Events at the Periphery

Following reactivation, viral genomes are transported to the epithelial surface. How this happens is unknown, although it is presumed to occur by retrograde axonal spread. Once at the periphery, it may or may not cause a clinical recurrence. The factors determining whether active epithelial viral replication occurs may include the anatomical site infected, the amount of virus present, the rapidity of the host cell response (Notkins 1974; Lopez 1985), the competence of the immune system and the degree of epithelial cell differentiation; young, undifferentiated cells may be more susceptible to HSV infection, and local "traumatic events" may increase the number of young undifferentiated cells (Hill et al. 1984).

The possibility that local traumatic events may increase the susceptibility of epithelial cells to herpetic infections deserves further consideration. Firstly, irradiation, stripping of the skin with Cellotape, local applications of xylene, dimethyl sulphoxide, or retinoic acid, and ultraviolet light, all give rise transiently to an increase in undifferentiated (and hence more susceptible) cells in the epithelium (Harbour et al. 1983). In addition, these local traumatic events also induce large increases in the levels of prostaglandins E and F in the skin (Hill and Blyth 1976). It has been suggested that prostaglandins may act as local skin triggers through their known immunosuppressive action (Goldyne 1983), as well as possibly enhancing the susceptability of epithelial cells to HSV.

These observations suggest that HSV arrives intermittently at the epithelial surface and, depending upon the factors mentioned above, clinical lesions may be produced or the virus may be shed from an apparently intact epithelium.

Role of the Immune System in the Production and Maintenance of Latency

The exact role of the immune system in the production and maintenance of latency and in subsequent reactivation is unknown. As discussed in Chap. 1, non-specific immune mechanisms (NK cell activation and interferons) and cell-mediated immunity control the extent of spread during primary infection. The early spread of the virus to nerve axons suggests that it may be immunologically privileged very early in the natural history of the infection (Wildy 1985). The virus remains immunologically privileged during the subsequent retrograde axonal spread to the neurones, in its latent and reactivated state within the neurone and during its anterograde spread back to the periphery.

What is the nature of this immunological privilege? Because nerve cells and their axons are a closed system, lymphocytes are unable to penetrate, and therefore, unless viral antigens are expressed on the surface of the neurones, none of the cell-mediated immune mechanisms will be activated. As mentioned above, viral reactivation probably involves only low-level gene production and none of the viral antigens is expressed on the neuronal surface. It is possible that some lymphokines may penetrate cells but their role (if any) is unclear. Therefore it seems unlikely that the immune system is particularly important in establishing or maintaining latency or in the reactivation of latent virus.

In marked contrast (as outlined in Chap. 1) the immune system (particularly cell-mediated immunity) is vital in controlling reactivated virus at the periphery. As discussed in Chap. 5, individuals with depressed cell-mediated immunity develop severe, prolonged, and often more frequent local recurrences as well as running the risk of developing disseminated disease.

Cervical Carcinoma

Introduction

There is considerable evidence to suggest a possible association between HSV and carcinoma of the cervix. However, whether HSV is directly or indirectly involved in this association or whether it is an innocent bystander is yet to be determined.

Over recent years attention has focussed on another virus, the human papilloma virus (HPV) as the initiator or promoter of cervical cancer (Anonymous 1985). The molecular evidence implicating HPV types 16 and 18 is very compelling and has to some extent overshadowed the evidence for a role for HSV. None the less, there is still a large amount of information about HSV and its possible role in the causation of cancer of the cervix, and this will be considered in detail below. Unfortunately absolute proof may be obtained only when and if an effective vaccine is developed or an antiviral drug capable of eliminating latency is produced (Rapp and Howett 1984; see also Chap. 8).

Epidemiological Evidence

The epidemiological evidence linking cancer of the cervix and herpes comes mainly from serological surveys. As discussed in Chap. 7 the serological diagnosis of HSV is complicated by the diversity of assays, and the extensive cross-reactivity between HSV 1 and HSV 2. The newly described immunodot enzymic assays using monoclonal antibodies to type-specific glycoproteins (Lee et al. 1985, 1986; see also Chap. 7) have not yet been evaluated in large-scale surveys. The problem of controlling for other factors possibly associated with carcinoma of the cervix, for example:

Young age at first coitus

Multiple sexual partners

Early marriage

Multiple marriages

Partner(s) with multiple previous partners

Partner(s) with penile cancer

Smoking

Human papilloma virus

further complicates interpretation. Two types of seroepidemiological surveys have been conducted: (1) retrospective studies looking at patients with known cervical cancer and matching them to controls; and (2) prospective population-based studies, following large numbers of healthy women to see which factors are important in the subsequent development of cervical carcinoma.

If we look first at the retrospective studies, an overall picture emerges. This suggests that the prevalence of antibodies to HSV 2 is highest in women with cervical carcinoma, lower in those with carcinoma in situ (now termed cervical interepithelial neoplasia (CIN) grade III), and still lower in those with mild dysplasia (CIN I and II). Women with normal cervices have the lowest prevalence of HSV 2 antibodies (Adam et al. 1972; Catalano and Johnson 1971; Nahmias et al. 1970; Rawls et al. 1970, 1972, 1973; Rawls and Campione-Piccardo 1981; Rotkin 1973; Priden and Lilienfeld 1971).

A recent study from Rawls et al (1986) using logistic regression analysis showed that several factors were related to cervical cancer. These included multiple marriages, young age at first sexual intercourse, early age of first marriage or pregnancy, multiple marriages and antibodies to HSV 2. The best predictor was antibodies to HSV 2. Although there was a linear relationship between the occurrence of anti-HSV 2 antibodies and the incidence of cervical carcinoma, this was not true in some population groups, suggesting that either HSV 2 infection may be a co-variable with other factors, or the virus is solely responsible for the tumour in only a small proportion of cases.

Finally, a recent study from Denmark and Greenland is worthy of some consideration (Kjaer et al. 1988). In this study, two populations were investigated. The one in Greenland had a very high incidence of cervical cancer, the other in Denmark had a lower incidence. Indeed the incidence in Greenland is 5.7 times higher than that in Denmark. From each country, authors randomly selected 800 women between 29 and 39 years of age from a population register. They were able to include 586 (84.3%) of the 695 eligible women in Greenland and 661 (84.2%) of the 785 in Denmark. All women had a cervical smear, and a specimen for HPV DNA hybridisation and a serum sample for HSV antibodies were taken from each one. In the Greenland women (i.e. the population with the higher incidence of cervical cancer), HPV types 16 and 18 were detected less frequently than in the Danish women. In contrast antibodies to both HSV 1 and HSV 2 were significantly more common in the Greenland women.

The findings from the prospective studies are somewhat different. Two such studies have been done. The first from Prague (Vonka et al. 1984a, b, 1987) included 10 389 women volunteers, aged 25–45 years, selected from a register of electors. The authors carefully matched patients with cancer and those with CIN II and CIN III with controls. Factors controlled for included age, smoking, numbers of sexual partners, age of first intercourse and previous diathermo-electrocoagulation of the ectopic epithelium and transformation zone of the cervix. Using two different serological assays the authors were unable to show any correlation between cervical abnormalities and presence of HSV 2 antibodies.

The second prospective study was conducted in the USA on a group of women who had been exposed in utero to diethylstilboestrol (DES) (Adam et al. 1985). The women were followed for five to seven years, and examined regularly to detect any evidence of CIN or invasive carcinoma. Twenty-three with CIN II or III were detected. There were no cases of invasive cancer. The 23 cases of CIN were matched with controls of a similar age. Nine per cent of both groups had antibodies to HSV 2 at enrolment. However, 52% (12) of the 23 CINs and 22%

(5) of the 23 controls had HSV 1 antibodies ($P<0.05$). This study has a number of problems of interpretation. The numbers were very small, no case of invasive cancer was seen and the methods used to detect antibodies are less reliable than the newer techniques discussed above.

It is evident that the seroepidemiological argument is far from resolved. The retrospective studies suggest an association, but the prospective ones do not. The results of surveys using well-validated type-specific serological assays are awaited with interest.

Virological Evidence

Indirect Evidence

There are several indirect strands of virological evidence which point towards a possible link between HSV and cervical cancer. Firstly, animal herpes viruses have been implicated in the causation of several tumours: these include Marek's disease in chickens (Churchill and Biggs 1967; Nazerian et al. 1968), lymphoma in monkeys (Melendez et al. 1970, 1972; Wolfe et al. 1971) and Lücke's tumour (renal adenocarcinoma) in frogs (Granoff 1973). Secondly, in man there is evidence linking Burkitt's lymphoma and nasopharangeal carcinoma with EBV (a herpes group virus; Epstein et al. 1964). Final proof, however, awaits the development of a vaccine. Finally, the virus is known to infect the cervix at the squamocolumnar junction. Studies by Vesterinen et al. (1978) showed that productive cervical infection (as evidenced by intranuclear inclusions and giant cell formation) was more likely to affect the ectocervical cells than those of the endocervix. The former is the site where most tumours arise.

Transformation of Cells

In 1971 Duff and Rapp reported on the transformation of hamster cells in culture from normal to oncogenic phenotype as a result of infection irradiated (and hence partially inactivated) HSV 2. Since then several other studies have shown that irradiated HSV can transform various rodent cell lines (Darai and Munk 1973; Kutinova et al. 1973; Munyon et al. 1971). Human cells have not yet been transformed from normal to malignant phenotype, but transforming doses of virus has been shown to alter cell morphology.

In an attempt to identify which viral genes are responsible for transformation, several experiments using defined viral DNA fragments have been conducted. In 1981, Galloway and McDougall showed that a fragment of HSV 2 DNA (0.58–0.63 map units) designated BglII-N was capable of transforming rodent cells. It is of interest that this particular region of the viral genome had previously been shown to have transforming potential (Reyes et al. 1979). Later experiments with the BglII-N sequence showed that a 2.1 kb (1 kb $=10^3$ base-pairs) fragment from the left half and bounded by BamHI site was capable of transformation, (for a full explanation and gene map see Fig. 1 of Galloway and McDougall 1983). Although the 2.1 kb fragment was not retained, recent evidence suggests that a 227 base-pair fragment was (Galloway and McDougall 1983).

Another fragment on the right of the *Bgl*II-N fragment (between 0.41–0.58 map units) may also be involved (Jariwalla et al. 1980). Indeed it has been suggested that the region of the genome responsible for transformation may be a two-part sequence. The fragment on the left may be involved in the production of immortal lines and that on the right in the conversion from preneoplastic immortal lines to a tumorigenic state (Jariwalla et al. 1980, 1983; Aurelian 1984).

Two specific viral proteins designated ICP10 (also known as AG4) and ICP12 are expressed in the transformed cells (Manak et al. 1981; Strnad and Aurelian 1978; Smith and Aurelian 1979). Further experiments indicate that ICP10 may be the protein responsible for the acquisition and maintenance of anchorage-dependent tumorigenic lines (Aurelian 1984).

Animal Models

One of the problems with experiments in vivo is that HSV often causes disseminated infection in laboratory animals unless very low doses are given. In 1975 Nahmias et al. were able to demonstrate low-level (<4%) tumour development in baby hamsters inoculated with small numbers of live or inactivated HSV 2. The presence of virus could not be demonstrated in the tumour. More recent studies have shown that prolonged exposure of mouse cervix to inactivated HSV 2 results in dysplasia, microinvasion and even invasive disease (Wentz et al. 1981). Of particular interest are the subsequent experiments showing that pre-exposure vaccination against HSV 2 prevents the subsequent development of tumours in mouse cervix exposed to inactivated virus (Wentz et al. 1983).

Detection of Genetic Information from Cervical Tumours

Before looking at the more specific virological evidence, I will consider briefly the various mechanisms that may be involved in the causation of tumours by viruses, as this may help to unravel some of the complexities and apparent contradictions in the experimental data.

There are three basic mechanisms of viral oncogenesis. The first is by integration of viral oncogenes into host DNA. The second is by activation of host oncogenes either by cellular translocation to escape repressor mechanisms or by integration close to cellular oncogenes, with subsequent activation. With both of these mechanisms one would expect to find evidence of residual genome in the tumour. Finally, viruses may act as promoters of mutagens. This has been termed the "hit-and-run" mechanism (Fig. 2.2; see also Galloway and McDougall 1983). One would not expect to find evidence of viral genomes in tumours caused in this way.

If HSV is integrated into host DNA, one would expect to find evidence of HSV DNA or mRNA in cervical tumours. In 1972, Frenkel et al. using a DNA probe to the whole virus genome, were able to detect a segment of the HSV 2 genome at a concentration of 3.4 copies per cell, from cells derived from a cervical tumour. Other workers have not been able to repeat this work (Pagano 1975; Zur Hausen et al. 1974). More recently Galloway and McDougall (1983)

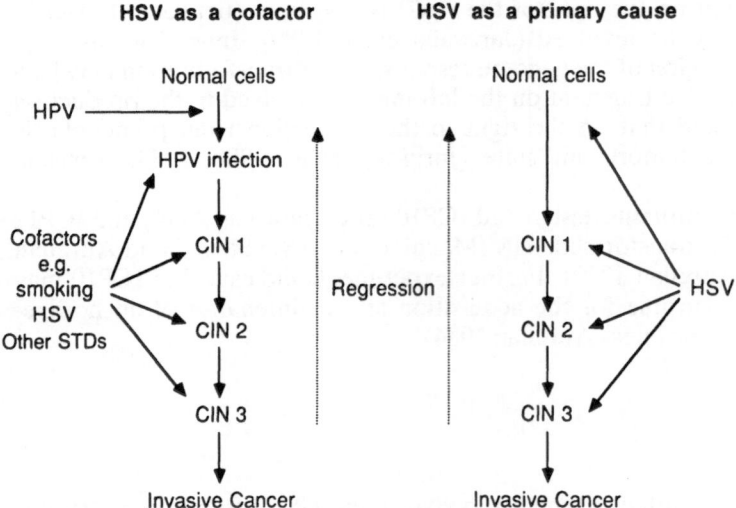

Fig. 2.2. Pathogenisis of cervical carcinoma, Two possible mechanisms: *HSV as a co-factor* and *HSV as a primary cause*. *STDs*, sexually-transmitted diseases; *HPV*, human papilloma virus; *CIN*, cervical intraepithelial neoplasia.

reported on the detection of viral DNA from three of nine cervical tumour biopsies. The probes they used were derived from HSV 2 DNA fragments.

In 1982 McDougall et al. published the results of experiments using in situ hybridisation to detect HSV mRNA in frozen sections from patients with invasive cancer, dysplasia and carcinoma in situ, and benign lesions including squamous metaplasia. HSV mRNA was present in 30% of the specimens from patients with cancerous or precancerous lesions, and was shown to span regions in the active HSV viral genome.

Three viral proteins have been identified in cervical cancer cells. These include two ICP10 and ICP12, both of which are expressed in HSV 2 transformed cells (see above) and a third protein designated ICSP 34/35. Aurelian et al. (1983) using a monospecific anti-ICP10 immunofluorescent stain were able to detect antigens in 90% of patients with invasive cancer or carcinoma in situ, in 70% of those with severe dysplasia, in 46% with mild dysplasia and in 10% of controls. A study where 209 patients with cervical carcinoma were followed prospectively indicated that 87 patients converted from being ICP10 seropositive prior to treatment to being ICP10 seronegative after. In addition, the patients who were seropositive throughout had a recurrence of their tumour (Aurelian et al. 1981).

ICP12 (also known as AG-e, ICSP 11/2 and VP143) (Dreesman et al. 1980; Flannery et al. 1977) is expressed in a small number of ICP10-positive cervical tumour cells (Aurelian et al. 1983). This antigen appears to induce a specific immune response in women with cervical cancer. Lymphocytes from 75% of patients with cervical cancer or dysplasia responded to ICP12 in a leukocyte migration assay, compared with only 13% of controls (Bell et al. 1978). The role of the third antigen ICSP 34/35 remains unknown (Dreesman et al. 1980).

Vulva Carcinoma

The number of women with squamous cell carcinoma in situ of the vulva is reported to be increasing (Japaze et al. 1977; Bender et al. 1980). As the majority of cases are under 40 years of age and HSV also is common in women of this age group, it has been postulated that the two might be related. Although this is an attractive hypothesis, there is only one study to back it up. In 1981 Kaufman et al. found herpes antigens, including ICP10 and ICP12, in the cells of nine out of ten patients with carcinoma in situ or severe dysplasia. Further work will be needed to validate these findings.

Conclusions

The possible association between HSV and genital tumours, in particular carcinoma of the cervix, remains an interesting but as yet unproven hypothesis. The seroepidemiological surveys and transformation experiments provide some circumstantial evidence, but the detection of HSV viral proteins in cervical cancer cells is more convincing. Final proof awaits the possible production of an HSV vaccine.

References

Adam E, Kaufman RH, Melnick JL, Levy AH, Rawls WE (1972) Seroepidemiologic studies of herpesvirus type 2 and carcinoma of the cervix III Houston Texas. Am J Epidemiol 96: 427–442

Adam E, Kaufman RH, Adler-Storthz K, Melnick JL, Dreesman GR (1985) A prospective study of association of herpes simplex virus and human papillomavirus infections with cervical neoplasia in women exposed to diethylstillboestrol in utero. Int J Cancer 35: 19–26

Anonymous (1985) Genital warts, human papillomavirus and cervical cancer. Lancet ii: 1045–1046

Aurelian L (1984) Herpes simplex virus type 2 and cervical cancer. Clin Dermatol 2: 90–99

Aurelian L, Kessler II, Rosensheim NB, Barbour G (1981) Viruses and gynaecologic cancers: herpesvirus protein (ICP10/AG-4a) cervical tumor antigens that fulfill the criteria for a marker of carcinogenicity. Cancer 48: 455–471

Aurelian L, Smith CC, Klacsmann TT, Gupta PK, Frost JK (1983) Expression and cellular compartmentalisation of a herpes simplex virus type 2 protein (ICP10) in productively infected and cervical tumour cells. Cancer Invest 1: 301–313

Baringer JR, Swoveland P (1974) Persistent herpes simplex virus infection in rabbit trigeminal ganglia. Lab Invest 30: 230–240

Becker Y, Shtram Y, Hadar J, et al. (1984) Herpes simplex virus type 1 thymidine kinase gene controls virus pathogenesis and latency in the nervous system. In: Kohn A, Fuchs P (eds) Mechanism of viral pathogenesis. Matinus Nijhoff, Boston, MA, pp 293-308

Bell RB, Aurelian L, Cohen G (1978) Proteins of herpesvirus type 2. IV. Leukocyte inhibition responses to type-common antigens in cervix cancer and recurrent herpetic infections. Cell Immunol 41: 86–102

Bender ME, Katz HI, Posalaky Z (1980) Carcinoma in situ of the genitalia. JAMA 243: 145–147

Blyth WA, Harbour DA, Hill TJ (1984) Pathogenesis of zosteriform spread of herpes simplex virus in the mouse. J Gen Virol 65: 1477–1486

Cantin EM, Puga A, Notkins AL (1984) Molecular biology of herpes simplex virus latency. In: Notkins AL, Oldstone MBA (eds) Concepts in viral pathogenesis, Springer, Berlin, Heidelberg, New York, pp 172–177

Catalano LW, Johnson LD (1971) Herpes virus antibody and carcinoma in situ of the cervix. JAMA 217: 447–450

Churchill AE, Biggs PM (1967) Agent of Marek's disease in tissue culture. Nature 215: 528–530

Corey L, Adams HG, Brown ZA, Holmes KK (1983) Genital herpes simplex virus infections: clinical manifestations, course and complications. Ann Intern Med 98: 958–972

Croen KD, Ostrove JM, Dragovic LJ, Smialek JE, Straus SE (1987) Latent herpes simplex virus in human trigeminal ganglia. Detection of an immediate early gene "anti-sense" transcript by in situ hybridisation. N Engl J Med 317: 1427–1432

Darai G, Munk K (1973) Human embryonic lung cells abortively infected with herpesvirus hominis type 2 show some properties of cell transformation. Nature New Biol 241: 268–269

Doerfler W (1981) DNA methylation – a regulatory signal in eukaryotic gene expression. J Gen Virol 57: 1–20

Dreesman GR, Burk J, Ada E, et al. (1980) Expression of herpesvirus induced antigens in human cervical cancer. Nature 283: 591–593

Duff R, Rapp F (1971) Oncogenic transformation of hamster cells after exposure to herpes simplex virus type 2. Nature New Biol 233: 43–50

Epstein MA, Achong BG, Barr YM (1964) Virus particles in cultured lymphoblasts from Burkitt's lymphoma. Lancet i: 702–703

Field HJ, Darby G (1980) Pathogenicity in mice of strains of herpes simplex virus which are resistant to acyclovir in vitro and in vivo. Antimicrob Agents Chemother 17: 209–216

Flannery V, Courtney R, Schaffer P (1977) Expression of an early, nonstructural antigen of herpes simplex virus in cells transformed in vitro by herpes simplex virus. J Virol 21: 284–291

Frenkel N, Roizman B, Cassai E, Nahmias A (1972) A DNA fragment of herpes simplex 2 and its transcription in human cervical cancer tissue. Proc Nat Acad Sci USA 69: 3734–3789

Galloway DA, McDougall JK (1981) Transformation of rodent cells by a cloned DNA fragment of herpes simplex virus type 2. J Virol 38: 749–760

Galloway DA, McDougall JK (1983) The oncogenic potential of herpes simplex viruses: evidence for a hit and run mechanism. Nature 302: 21–24

Galloway DA, Fenoglio C, Shevchuk M, McDougall JK (1979) Detection of herpes simplex RNA in human sensory ganglia. Virology 95: 265–268

Galloway DA, Fenoglio C, McDougall JK (1982) Limited transcription of the herpes virus genome when latent in human sensory ganglia. J Virol 41: 686–691

Goldyne ME (1983) Eicosanoids and immunoregulation. Rec Adv Clin Immuno 3: 9–36

Goodpasture EW (1929) Herpetic infection with a special reference to involvement of the nervous system. Medicine (Baltimore) 8: 223–243

Granoff A (1973) Herpesvirus and the Lücke's tumor. Cancer Res 33: 1431–1433

Green MT, Courtney RJ, Dunkel EC (1981) Detection of an immediate early herpes simplex type 1 polypeptide in trigeminal ganglia from latently infected animals. Infect Immun 34: 987–992

Guinan ME, MacCalman J, Kern ER, Overall JC, Spruance SL (1981) The course of untreated recurrent genital herpes simplex infection in 27 women. New Engl J Med 304: 759–763

Harbour DA, Hill TJ, Blyth WA (1983) Recurrent herpes simplex in the mouse. Inflammation in the skin and activation of virus in the ganglia following peripheral inoculation. J Gen Virol 64: 1491–1498

Hill TJ (1984) Herpes simplex virus latency. In: Roizman B (ed) The herpesvirus, vol 3, New York, Plenum Press, pp 175–240

Hill TJ, Blyth WA (1976) An alternative theory of herpes simplex recurrence and a possible role for prostaglandins. Lancet i: 397–399

Hill TJ, Altmann DM, Blyth WA, Harbour DA, Whitby A (1984) Herpes simplex virus latency. Clin Dermatol 2: 46–55

Japaze H, Garcia-Bunuel R, Woodruff JD (1977) Primary vulvar neoplasia: a review of in situ and invasive carcinoma 1935–1972. Obstet Gynecol 49: 404–411

Jariwalla RJ, Aurelian L, Ts'o POP (1980) Tumorigenic transformation induced by a specific fragment of herpes simplex virus type 2 DNA. Proc Natl Acad Sci USA 77: 2279–2283

Jariwalla RJ, Aurelian L, Ts'o POP (1983) Immortalization and neoplastic transformation of normal diploid cells by various DNA fragments of herpes simplex virus type 2 (HSV 2). Proc Natl Acad Sci USA 80: 5902–5906

Joseph BS, Oldstone MB (1974) Expression of selected antigens on the surface of cultured neuronal cells. Brain Res 80: 421–434

Kastoukoff L, Long C, Doherty PC, Wroblewska Z, Koprowski H (1981) Isolation of virus from brain after immune suppression of mice with latent herpes simplex. Nature 291: 432–433

Kaufman RH, Dreesman GR, Burek J, et al. (1981) Herpesvirus-induced antigen in squamous cell carcinoma in situ of the vulva. N Engl J Med 305: 483–488

Kjaer SK, De Villiers EM, Haugaard BJ, et al. (1988) Human Papillomavirus herpes simplex virus and cervical cancer incidence in Greenland and Denmark. A population-based cross-sectional study. Int J Cancer 44: 518–524

Kreutzberg GW (1982) Acute neuronal reaction to injury. In: Nicholls JG (ed) Repair and regeneration of the nervous system. Springer, Berlin, Heidelberg, New York, pp 71-89

Kristensson K (1978) Retrograde transport to macromolecules in axons. Annu Rev Pharmacol Toxicol 18: 97–110

Kutinova L, Vonka V, Broucek J (1973) Increased oncogenicity and synthesis of herpesvirus antigens in hamster cells exposed to herpes simplex type 2 virus. J Natl Cancer Inst 50: 759–766

Lafferty WE, Coombs RW, Benedetti J, Critchlow C, Corey L (1987) Recurrences after oral and genital herpes simplex virus infection. Influence of site of infection and viral type. New Engl J Med 316: 1444–1449

Lee FK, Colman RM, Pereira L, Bailey PD, Tatsuno M, Nahmias AJ (1985) Detection of herpes simplex virus type 2-specific antibody with glycoprotein G. J Clin Microbiol 22: 641–644

Lee FK, Pereira L, Griffin C, Reid E, Nahmias A J (1986) A novel glycoprotein for detection of herpes simplex virus type 1 specific antibodies. J Virol Methods 14: 111-118

Lieberman AR (1971) The axon reaction. A review of the principle features of perikaryal responses to axon injury. Int Rev Neurobiol 14: 49–124

Lieberman AR (1974) Some factors affecting retrograde neuronal responses to axonal lesions. In: Bellaires R, Gray E G (eds) Essays on the nervous system, Clarendon Press, Oxford, pp 71–105

Lindahl T, Adams A, Bjursell G, et al. (1976) Covalently closed circular duplex DNA of Epstein–Barr virus in a human lymphoid cell line. J Mol Biol 102: 511–530

Lofgren KW, Stevens JG, Marsden HS, Subak-Sharpe JH (1977) Temperature-sensitive mutants of herpes simplex virus differ in the capacity to establish latent infection in mice. Virology 76: 440–443

Lopez C (1985) Natural resistance mechanisms in herpes simplex virus infections. In: Roizman B, Lopez C (eds) The herpesvirus: immunobiology and prophylaxis of human herpesvirus infections, vol 4, New York, Plenum Press, pp 37–68

Lycke E, Kristensson K, Svennalholm B, Vahlne A, Ziegler R (1984) Uptake and transport of herpes simplex virus in neurites of rat dorsal root dorsal ganglia cells in culture. J Gen Virol 65: 55–64

Manak MM, Smith C, Aurelian L (1981) Focus formation and neoplastic transformation by herpes simplex virus type 2 inactivated intracellularly by BUdR and near UV light. J Virol 40: 289–300

McDougall JK, Crum CP, Fenoglio CM, Goldstein LC, Galloway DA (1982). Herpesvirus-specific RNA and protein in carcinoma of the uterine cervix. Proc Natl Acad Sci USA 79: 3853–3857

McLennan JL, Darby G (1980) Herpes simplex virus latency: the cellular location of virus in dorsal root ganglia and the fate of the infected cell following virus activation. J Gen Virol 51: 233–243

Melendez LV, Hunt RD, Daniel MD, Fraser CEO, Garcia FG, Williamson ME (1970) Lethal reticuloproliferative disease induced in Cebus albifrons monkeys by herpesvirus saimiri. Int J Cancer 6: 431–435

Melendez LV, Hunt RD, King NW, et al. (1972) Herpesvirus ateles a new lymphoma virus of monkeys. Nature New Biol 235: 182–184

Mindel A, Sutherland S (1983) Genital herpes – the disease and its treatment including intravenous acyclovir. J Antimicrob Chemother 12 [suppl B]: 51–59

Mindel A, Coker DM, Faherty A, Williams P (1988) Recurrent genital herpes: clinical and virological features in men and women. Genitourin Med 64: 103–106

Munyon W, Kraiselburd E, Davis D, Mann J (1971) Transfer of thymidine kinase to thymidine kinaseless L cells by infection with ultraviolet irradiated herpes simplex virus. J Virol 7: 813–820

Nahmias AJ, Josey WE, Naib ZM, Luce CF, Guest B (1970) Antibodies to herpesvirus hominis types 1 and 2 in humans. II. Women with cervical cancer. Am J Epidemiol 91: 547–552

Nahmias AJ, Del Buono I, Ibrahim I (1975) Antigenic relationship between herpes simplex viruses; human cervical cancer and HSV associated with hamster tumours. IARC Sci Publ 11: 309–313

Nazerian K, Solomon JJ, Witter RL, et al. (1968) Studies on the etiology of Marek's disease. II. Finding of a herpes virus in cell cultures. Proc Soc Exp Biol Med 127: 177–182

Notkins AL (1974) Immune mechanisms by which the spread of viral infections is stopped. Cell Immunol 11: 478–483

Openshaw H, Sekizawa T, Wohlenberg C, Notkins AL (1981) The role of immunity in latency and

reactivation of herpes simplex viruses. In: Nahmias A J, Dowdle W R, Schinazi RF (eds) The
    human herpesvirus. An interdisciplinary perspective. Elsevier, New York, pp 289–296
Overall JC Jr (1984) Dermatologic viral diseases. In: Galasso GJ, Merigan TC and Buchanan RA
    (eds) Antiviral agents and viral diseases of man, 2nd edn. Raven Press, New York, pp 247–312
Pagano JS (1975) Diseases and mechanisms of persistent DNA virus infection: latency and cellular
    transformation. J Infect Dis 132: 209–223
Price RW (1979) 6-Hydroxydopamine potentiates acute herpes virus infection of the superior
    cervical ganglion in mice. Science 205: 518–520
Price RW (1985) Herpes simplex virus latency: adaptation to the peripheral nervous system. Cancer
    Invest 3: 389–603
Price RW, Khan A (1981) Resistance of peripheral autonomic nerves to in vivo productive infection
    by herpes simplex virus mutants deficient in thymidine kinase activity. Infect Immun 34: 571–580
Price RW, Schmitz J (1979) Route of infection, systemic host resistance and integrity of ganglionic
    axons influence acute and latent herpes simplex virus infections of the superior cervical ganglion.
    Infect Immun 23: 373–383
Priden H, Lilienfeld AM (1971) Carcinoma of the cervix in Jewish women in Israel 1960–67. An
    epidemiological survey. Israel J Med Sci: 1465–1470
Puga A, Rosenthal JD, Openshaw H, Notkins AL (1978) Herpes simplex virus DNA and mRNA
    sequences in acutely and chronically infected trigeminal ganglia of mice. Virology 89: 102–111
Puga A, Cantin EM, Wohlenberg C, Openshaw H, Notkins AL (1984) Different sizes of restriction
    endonuclease fragments from the terminal repetitions of the herpes simplex virus type 1 genome
    latent in the trigeminal ganglia of mice. J Gen Virol: 65, 437–444
Rapp F, Howett MK (1984) Herpesvirus and cancer. In: Notkins AL, Oldstone MBA (Eds)
    Concepts in viral pathogens. Springer, Berlin, Heidelberg, New York, pp 300–306
Rawls WE, Campione-Piccardo J (1981) Epidemiology of herpes simplex viruses type 1 and type 2
    infections In: Nahmias AJ, Dowdle WR, Schinazi F (eds) The human herpesvirus. Elsevier, New
    York, pp 137–152
Rawls WE, Iwamoto K, Adam E, Melnick JL (1970) Herpesvirus type 2 antibodies and carcinoma of
    the cervix. Lancet ii: 1142
Rawls WE, Adam E, Melnick JL (1972) Geographic variation in the association of antibodies to
    herpesvirus type 12 and carcinoma of the cervix. In: de The' G, Biggs P M, Payne L N (eds)
    Oncogenesis and herpes virus. International Agency for Research on Cancer, WHO, Lyons,
    pp 424–427
Rawls WE, Adam E, Melnick JL (1973) An analysis of seroepidemiological studies of herpes virus
    type 2 and cancer of the cervix. Cancer Res 33: 1477–1482
Rawls WE, Lavery C, Marrett LD, et al. (1986) Comparison of risk factors for cervical cancer in
    different populations. Int J Cancer 37: 537–546
Reeves WC, Corey L, Adams HG, Vontver LA, Holmes KK (1981) Risk or recurrence after first
    episode of genital herpes. Relation to HSV type and antibody response. New Engl J Med 305:
    315–319
Reyes GR, La Femina R, Hayward SD, Hayward GS (1979) Morphological transformation by DNA
    fragments of human herpes viruses: evidence for two distinct transforming regions in HSV 1 and
    HSV 2 and lack of correlation with biochemical transfer of the thymidine kinase gene. Cold
    Spring Harb Symp Quant Biol 44: 629–641
Rock DL, Fraser NW (1983) Detection of HSV-1 genome in cerebral nervous system of latently
    infected mice. Nature 302: 523–525
Rotkin ID (1973) A comparison review of key epidemiological studies in cervical cancer related to
    current searches for transmissible agents. Cancer Res 33: 1353–1367
Simmons A, Nash AA (1984) Zosteriform species of herpes simplex virus as a model of recrudence
    and its use to investigate the role of immune cells in prevention of recurrent disease. J Virol 52:
    816–821
Smith CC, Aurelian L (1979) Proteins of herpesvirus: characterisation of two viral proteins in a virus
    specific antigenic fraction. Virology 98: 255–260
Spruance SL, Overall JC, Kern ER, Krueger GC, Pliam V, Miller W (1977) The natural history of
    recurrent herpes simplex labialis. New Engl J Med 297: 69–75
Stevens JG, Wagner EK, Devi-Rao GB, Cook ML, Feldman LT (1987) RNA complementary to a
    herpesvirus gene in RNA is prominent in latently infected neurones. Science 235: 1056–1058
Strnad B, Aurelian L (1978) Proteins of herpesvirus type 2. III. Isolation and immunologic
    characterisation of a large molecular weight viral protein. Virology 87: 401–415
Sutherland S, Morgan B, Mindel A, Chan WL (1986) Typing and subtyping of herpes simplex
    isolates by monoclonal fluorescence. J Med Virol 18: 235–245

Tedder RS, Briggs M, Cameron CH, Honess R, Robertson D, Whittle H (1987) A novel lymphotropic herpesvirus. Lancet ii: 390–392

Tenser RB, Miller RL, Rapp F (1979) Trigeminal ganglion infection by thymidine kinase negative mutants of herpes simplex virus. Science 204: 915–917

Tenser RB, Ressel S, Dunstan ME (1981) Herpes simplex virus thymidine kinase expression in trigeminal ganglion infection: correlation of enzyme activity with ganglion virus titre and evidence of in vivo complementation. Virology 112: 328–341

Vahlne A, Nyström B, Sandberg M, Hamburger A, Lycke E (1978) Attachment of herpes simplex virus to neurones and glial cells. J Gen Virol 40: 359–371

Vesterinen E, Purola E, Saksela E, Leinikki P (1978) Clinical and virological findings in patients with cytologically diagnosed gynecologic herpes simplex infections. Acta Cytol (Baltimore) 21: 199–205

Vonka V, Kaňka J, Jeliňek J, et al. (1948a) Prospective study on the relationship between cervical neoplasia and herpes simplex type-2 virus. I: Epidemiological characteristics. Int J Cancer 33: 49–60

Vonka V, Kaňka J, Hirsch I, et al. (1948b) Prospective study on the relationship between cervical neoplasia and herpes simplex virus. II. Herpes simplex type 2 antibody presence in sera taken at enrolment. Int J Cancer 33: 61–66

Vonka V, Kaňka J, Roth Z (1987) Herpes simplex type 2 virus and cervical neoplasia. Advan Cancer Res 48: 149–191

Watson K, Stevens JG, Cook ML, Subak-Sharpe JH (1980) Latency competence of thirteen HSV 1 temperature sensitive mutants. J Gen Virol 49: 149–159

Wentz WB, Reagan W, Fu JS, Haggie AD, Anthony DD (1981) Experimental studies of carcinogenesis of the uterine cervix in mice. Gynecol Oncol 12: S90–S98

Wentz WB, Haggie AD, Anthony DP, Reagan JW (1983) Prevention of herpes simplex virus type 2 (HSV-2) induced cervical carcinoma in mice by pre-expansive immunization against HSV-2. In: Abstracts of paper presented at an international herpes virus workshop, p 196.

Wildy P (1985) Herpes viruses: a background. Brit Med Bull 41: 339–344

Wolfe LG, Falk LA, Deinhardt F (1971) Oncogenicity of herpesvirus saimiri in marmoset monkeys. J Natl Cancer Inst 47: 1145–1162

Yamamoto H, Walz MA, Notkins AL (1977) Viral specific thymidine kinase in sensory ganglia of mice infected with herpes simplex virus. Virology 76: 866–869

Youssoufian H, Mulder C, Hammer SM, Hirsch MS (1982) Methylation of the viral genome in an in vitro model of herpes simplex virus latency. Proc Natl Acad Sci USA 79: 2207–2210

Zur Hausen H, Schulte-Holthausen H, Wolf H, Dorries K, Eggar H (1974) Attempts to detect virus specific DNA in human tumours. II. Nucleic acid hybridisations with complementary RNA of human herpes group viruses. Int J Cancer 13: 657–664

Chapter 3

Epidemiology

Introduction

Infections with HSV 1 and 2 are amongst the commonest human viral diseases. However, the majority of individuals exposed to these viruses are asymptomatic, which makes epidemiological studies difficult. One of the fundamental biological properties of HSV (and other human viruses of the herpes group – varicella zoster, cytomegalovirus and Epstein–Barr virus) is the ability to establish latency following the initial infection. This ability (discussed in detail in Chap. 2) has an important bearing on the epidemiology of herpes infections, in that latent virus may periodically reactivate giving rise to clinical illness or asymptomatic, but none the less infectious, viral excretion.

Dowdle et al. (1967) first discovered that there were two distinct HSV viruses. It was believed that HSV 1 caused disease above the waist, and HSV 2 that below. However, this is now known to be an over simplification and both viral types can cause all the clinical syndromes. An additional problem in trying to unravel the complex epidemiology of HSV infection is that although patients exposed to HSV develop anti-HSV antibodies there is considerable antigenic cross-reactivity between HSV 1 and HSV 2. Indeed, until recently there was no available test which accurately and reliably differentiated between the two viral types (see Chap. 7). Epidemiological surveys (particularly those done in the late 1960s and early 1970s) need to be viewed with these problems in mind.

Transmission

Infection occurs when susceptible individuals are exposed to infectious virus during close personal contact, including mouth to mouth, genital to genital, mouth to genital, genital to anal, or mouth to anal contact. The incubation period is 2 to 14 days. Humans are the sole reservoirs of HSV infection.

Transmission occurring from individuals with obvious clinical herpes is well documented, although patients with active cold sores or genital herpes are often aware of the infectious nature of their complaint and many probably avoid interpersonal contact at that time. Infection can also come from patients with no apparent herpetic lesions. Asymptomatic herpes or inapparent viral excretion can occur in two situations. Firstly, patients with clinical herpes can shed virus asymptomatically from time to time. (Studies in women with recurrent genital herpes have shown that HSV can be isolated from 4%–14% of them during periods when they are asymptomatic (Guinan et al. 1981; Adam et al. 1980; Rattray et al. 1978).) The second group of patients are those who have never had clinical herpes and are yet found to shed virus asymptomatically. Viral shedding of this type has been documented from the saliva of 1%–5% of adults (Herrmann 1967; Lindgren et al. 1968) and 18%–20% of young children (Buddingh et al. 1953; Cesario et al. 1969), and the genital tract of 1%–15% of women (Vesterinen et al. 1979; Centifanto et al. 1971; Rawls et al. 1971; Baker and Plotkin 1979; Adam et al. 1980) and occasionally from that of males (Deardourff et al. 1974). All of these studies almost certainly underestimate the true incidence of asymptomatic viral excretion, because in most cases only a single specimen was taken.

In an attempt to answer how often patients acquired infection from individuals who were unaware that they were infected, a study evaluated 66 source contacts of patients with first-episode genital herpes. Only 17 (26%) were aware that they had herpes at the time of transmission (Mertz et al. 1985). In addition to the patients who knew they had herpes, the authors identified three groups who were able to transmit herpes unknowingly. Firstly, there were truly asymptomatic patients; secondly, there were those with complaints which they were unaware were herpes; and finally there were patients with asymptomatic but none the less clinically apparent lesions.

Studies from Nigeria and India have shown that up to 50% of children aged 1–10 years have antibodies to HSV 2 (Sogbetun et al. 1979; Seth et al. 1981), and it has been suggested that inanimate objects (e.g. bedclothes) could be a potential source of infection, particularly in conditions of high humidity and overcrowding. These studies ignore the problem of serological cross-reactivity between HSV 1 and 2. It is, indeed, equally plausible that some HSV 2 infections are contracted by non-sexual, but physical, contact in those conditions. The non-venereal treponematoses (e.g. yaws, bejal, pinta and non-venereal syphilis) are transmitted in this way (Douglas and Corey 1983). What other evidence is there that HSV can be transmitted by inanimate objects? There is a handful of case reports suggesting that in some children genital HSV is not sexually transmitted (Scott et al. 1952; Krugman 1952; Nahmias et al. 1968). Although shared towels or bed linen are a possible source of infection, a much more likely explanation is close non-sexual physical contact with an infected individual. A nosocomial outbreak of HSV was blamed on fomites (Linneman et al. 1975). In this outbreak, two infants admitted to the same hospital room, within a couple of days of each other contracted neonatal herpes. Restriction endonuclease analysis (see Chap. 7) showed that isolates from the two cases were identical. The most plausible explanation for this outbreak is a common source contact, perhaps one of the medical or nursing personnel with an asymptomatic infection (the role of asymptomatic transmission is discussed above), not infected bed linen, clothing or towels.

Several laboratory studies have documented that HSV in infective titres can survive in water, on moist cloth and on plastic surfaces for several hours under conditions of high humidity and temperature (Montefiore et al. 1980; Nerurkar et al. 1983; Larson and Bryson 1982; Turner et al. 1982). Douglas and Corey (1983) postulated that several hurdles would need to be overcome if transmission was to occur via such inanimate objects. These include inoculation of infected material in sufficient titres from a lesion on to the appropriate surface, contact with a susceptible individual, deposition on to an epidermal or mucosal surface and mechanical friction to aid infection. Although each of these events is possible, the overall sequences makes it extremely unlikely. It is evident that fomites can hardly ever be implicated in the transmission of herpes, and most "sporadic" cases occur as a result of contact with someone who has an inapparent infection.

Oral Infections

The total number of people infected with oral herpes, either asymptomatic or symptomatic, is unknown. Overall (1984) has estimated that there are half a million new cases of primary gingivostomatitis each year in the USA and that there are 98 million infected individuals currently in that country. If these estimates are correct, then the number of infected individuals throughout the world is likely to run into hundreds of millions.

There are very few studies looking at the incidence of primary oral herpes. A small study conducted in a children's home in Kansas, USA, showed that only 8 of 70 seronegative children seroconverted (six with clinically apparent gingivostomatitis) during a 6-year study (Cesario et al. 1969). A large study involving 14 000 Yugoslavian children aged between 0 and 9 years showed that the annual incidence of symptomatic oral herpes was 1.4%. Of these children, 13% had suffered from a symptomatic infection by the age of 9. The incidence of inapparent seroconversion was not reported (Juretic 1966). The majority of oral infections are due to HSV 1; however, it is likely that with the growing popularity of orogenital sexual contact type 2 infection of the lips and oropharynx has already become more common.

Seroepidemiological surveys conducted in various population groups suggest that the acquisition of antibodies to HSV 1 (presumed to be the major cause of oral HSV) is related to age and socio-economic status (Nahmias et al. 1970; Rawls et al. 1969; Black et al. 1974). Amongst American aboriginal Indians, over 50% have antibodies to HSV by the age of 5 years, 80% by the age of 10, and 95% by the age of 15. In comparison, only 20% of middle-class Americans have antibodies by age 5 and the 50% mark is not reached until age 25. The reason for this difference is probably related to living standards. Amongst poor people there is more close interpersonal contact because of crowded living conditions and lower standards of hygiene.

Of patients with a first attack of oral herpes, 20%–45% will suffer from a recurrence (Ship et al. 1967; Embil et al. 1975; Young et al. 1976). About a quarter of these patients will have more than two episodes per year. The reasons for reactivation are poorly understood (see Chap. 2). However, a variety of factors is thought to be important:

Local trauma
  Ultraviolet light
  Wind
  Other (e.g. chemical, local abrasions, etc.)
Concurrent infections
Local dental or surgical procedures
Viral type HSV 1 > HSV 2
? Menstruation
? Stress

A recent study by Lafferty et al. (1987) showed that patients with orolabial infection due to HSV 2 were less likely to recur than those with HSV 1. These findings will require confirmation, as all the patients were adults, all had acquired their infections through sexual contact and all had simultaneous infections in the genital area with virus of the same type. This study does confirm the clinical impression that orolabial herpes recurs less frequently than genital herpes (see below).

Although most cases occur as a result of sporadic person-to-person contact, outbreaks may occasionally be attributable to a specific source. A report indicated that 20 people developed primary gingivostomatitis over a 4-week period as a result of contact with a dental hygienist who had a herpetic whitlow (Manzella et al. 1984). Fortunately, outbreaks of this sort appear to be uncommon.

Genital Infections

The majority of genital infections are caused by HSV 2. However, there is considerable geographical variation in the prevalence of HSV 1 infections (Table 3.1). There are even a few studies where the majority of infections were caused by HSV 1 (Chang et al. 1974; Willmott and Muir 1978; Barton et al. 1982; Mindel et al. 1987). The reason for this is probably related to the popularity of oral-genital sexual activity in different communities.

Genital herpes was first reported from sexually transmitted disease clinics in the United Kingdom in 1972, when 4500 cases were reported (Genital herpes simplex 1972–86, unpublished report from Communicable Disease Surveillance Centre, 1988). The number of cases has increased substantially and by 1984 the number reported was 19 869. Just under half the cases have occurred in females (Fig.3.1). Although the sexual orientation of males is not reported, a recent study from London showed that 20% of patients with genital herpes were homosexual (Hindley and Adler 1985). Since 1984 the situation has changed. There has been a levelling off in the number of males and a marginal decrease in the number of females, perhaps reflecting increased condom use since the advent of the human immunodeficiency virus (HIV) epidemic. Genital herpes in

Table 3.1. Percentage of genital herpes caused by HSV 1

	Females	Males	Sex unknown	Clinical status	Reference
USA	4	0	—	NK	Nahmias et al. 1969
	13	—	—	NK	Kaufman et al. 1973
	—	—	52	NK	Chang et al. 1974
	—	—	19	NK	Brown et al. 1979
	37	—	—	NK	Kalinyak et al. 1979
	40	—	—	NK	McCaughtry et al. 1982
	—	—	14	P	Corey et al. 1982
	—	—	10	FE	Bryson et al. 1983
	—	—	7	FE }	Corey et al. 1983
	—	—	2	R }	
	—	26	—	NK	Docherty et al. 1984
	—	—	0	R	Douglas et al. 1984
	—	—	26	P }	Mertz et al. 1984
	—	—	3	FE }	
	6	1	—	R	Luby et al. 1984
UK	31	13	—	P	Peutherer et al. 1982
	—	—	52	NK	Willmott and Mair 1978
	53	86	—	P }	Barton et al. 1982
	50	60	—	R }	
	—	—	16	FE	Thin et al. 1983
	—	—	45	P }	Mindel and Sutherland 1983
	—	—	25	FE }	
	—	—	34	FE }	Kinghorn et al. 1983
	—	—	20	R }	
	25	—	—	FE	Mindel et al. 1986
	—	—	51	FE	Mindel et al. 1987
Sweden	12	3	—	NK	Jeansson and Molin 1974
France	22	9	—	NK	Tardieu and Friedel 1983
Canada	23	12	—	NK	Anonymous 1983
Israel	—	—	10	NK	Leventon–Kriss et al. 1983
Japan	40	—	—	NK	Kawana et al. 1982
Australia	15	5	—	NK	Anonymous 1981
New Zealand	—	—	11	NK	Tobias and Herman 1983

NK, not known; P, primary; FE, first episode; R, recurrence

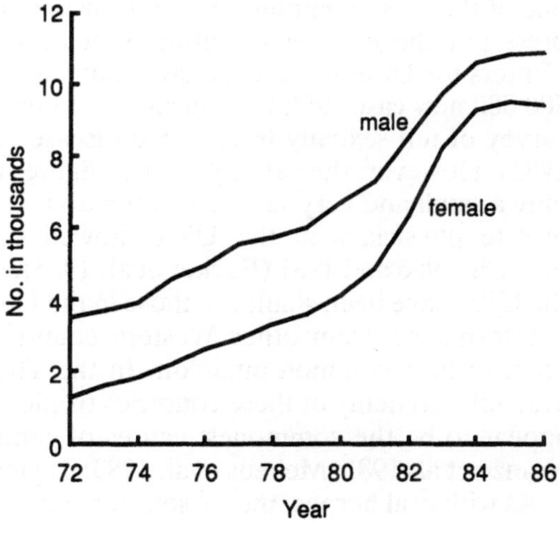

Fig. 3.1. Reported cases of genital herpes from sexually transmitted disease clinics in the United Kingdom, 1972–1986. (From unpublished report from Communicable Disease Surveillance Centre, 1988.)

Table 3.2. Reported cases of sexually transmitted
diseases, United Kingdom 1986

Non-specific genital infection	175 112
Genital warts	75 995
Candidiasis	68 928
Gonorrhoea	45 817
Genital herpes	20 315
Trichomoniasis	15 077
Pediculosis pubis	10 522
Molluscum contagiosum	3 044
Syphilis	2 203
Scabies	1 932
Other treponemal diseases	537
Chancroid	51
Lymphogranuloma venereum	46
Granuloma inguinale	20
Other conditions	
Not requiring treatment	154 076
Requiring treatment	128 548
Total	702 223

Data from unpublished report from Communicable
Disease Surveillance Centre, 1988.

the UK is now the fifth commonest diagnosis from sexually transmitted disease
clinics (Table 3.2). The apparent increase in genital herpes over recent years
may be due partly to increased publicity about the disease and current antiviral
treatments, the inclusion of both primary and recurrent cases in clinic returns
(Hindley and Adler 1985) and the increased use of viral cultures for diagnosis.
The size of the increase, however, suggests that a considerable part of it is
real.

The number of patients with genital herpes in other countries is less clear. In
the USA no accurate national data are available. However, herpes is said to be
one of the most common sexually transmitted diseases. Estimates in the popular
press put the number of sufferers at between 2 million and 20 million. The
Centers for Disease Control have estimated that there are between 300 000 and
500 000 new cases of herpes each year in the USA. These figures are based on a
survey of ten sexually transmitted disease clinics (Centers for Disease Control
1982). However, the validity of these figures is questionable as these clinics serve
only a small and very selected population. A recent review of patients attending
private physicians in the USA showed that attendances increased 7½-fold
between 1966 and 1981 (Becker et al. 1985), suggesting that the increases seen in
the USA have been similar to those in the UK.

Information from other Western countries is scarce, although herpes does
seem to be a common infection. In the Third World very little information is
available. In many of these countries tropical infections, in particular chancroid,
appear to be the commonest causes of genital ulceration (Duncan et al. 1981;
Nsanze et al. 1981; Meheus et al. 1983; Taylor et al. 1984).

As with oral herpes, the reasons for subsequent reactivation following the first attack of genital herpes have not been fully elucidated. However, several factors are known to be important:

Viral type HSV 2 > HSV 1

Local trauma
  Sexual intercourse
  Masturbation
Concurrent infections
Menstruation
?Stress

It is now well documented from several studies that patients with genital herpes due to HSV 2 recur earlier and suffer more frequent recurrences than patients with HSV 1 (Reeves et al. 1981; Mindel and Sutherland 1983; Lafferty et al. 1987). Indeed by the end of the first year virtually all patients with HSV 2 will have suffered from a recurrence, whereas only half of those with HSV 1 will have done so. It has also been documented that women recur less frequently than men and in female patients recurrences are more likely to occur around the time of menstruation (Mindel et al. 1988; Reeves et al. 1981; Guinan et al. 1981).

Ocular Herpes

The number of cases of ocular herpes occurring world-wide each year is unknown. However, estimates put the number of cases diagnosed yearly in the USA at 300 000, making ocular herpes the leading cause of corneal blindness (Pavan-Langston 1984; Kaufman 1978). The situation in other industrialised countries is likely to be similar. In the Third World the situation is largely unknown, but the condition is said to be becoming more common than previously (Darougar et al. 1985). The majority of ocular isolates are HSV 1 (Oh et al. 1985; Hanna et al. 1976). It is unknown whether asymptomatic or subclinical eye infection occurs.

The majority of primary infections occur in patients over the age of 15 (Darougar et al. 1985). Comparing the situation in recent years with that in the 1960s, the number of adolescents with primary ocular herpes seems to have increased, whilst the number of children under 15 years with the disease has decreased (Darougar et al. 1985; Patterson and Jones 1967). The reasons for this are unclear.

In patients with a first episode of eye disease there are two possible sources of infection, namely contact with another infected individual or reactivation of latent trigeminal ganglion infection (Dawson 1984). Patients exposed to HSV for the first time are likely to have systemic symptoms, including malaise, fever and a flu-like condition, whereas those with reactivated HSV are not (Darougar et al. 1985).

Up to a quarter of patients will suffer from a recurrence within the first year and a third within two years (Shuster et al. 1981); some patients have several recurrences per year (Bell et al. 1982). The majority of recurrences occur in the eye originally infected; however, up to 11% may occur in the opposite eye and 2% in both eyes (Bell et al. 1982). As with oral and genital HSV the reasons for recurrences are not well understood, although one study showed a seasonal variation, with more recurrences in winter (Bell et al. 1982). Bell et al. suggested that this was due to intercurrent upper respiratory tract viral infections.

Herpes Encephalitis and Disseminated Infections

HSV is estimated to be the commonest cause of fatal endemic encephalitis, as well as the commonest viral infection of the central nervous system in the USA (Corey and Spear 1986). Infection may be primary, particularly in children, or as a result of reactivation of pre-existing infection, which usually occurs in adults (Whitley et al. 1982). The number of subclinical or asymptomatic central nervous system infections is unknown. In adults, over 90% of isolates are HSV 1 positive (Whitley et al. 1977). There is no seasonal variation. Most cases occur in two age groups, patients aged 5 to 30 years and those over 50 years (Corey and Spear 1986).

Disseminated infections are almost always a result of reactivation of pre-existing latent infection in susceptible hosts (e.g. immunosuppressed patients or those with skin disease – see Chap. 5). Sporadic cases of disseminated HSV do apparently occur in patients with normal immunity.

Neonatal Infection

Neonatal herpes is not a notifiable disease and consequently the incidence of the infection is largely unknown. Studies in selected populations in America suggest that the incidence is anywhere between 2.6 to 50 per 100 000 live births (Nahmias et al. 1983; Sullivan-Bolyai et al. 1983), and in Seattle, WA, the incidence increased from 2.6 to 11.9 cases per 100 000 live births during the years 1966–1981 (Sullivan-Bolyai et al. 1983). In the United Kingdom the incidence is very much lower, probably in the neighbourhood of 1.6 to 1.8 cases per 100 000 live births.

Infection in the foetus or newborn infant may be acquired from several possible sources (Table 3.3). Foetal infection probably via transplacental transmission is exceptionally rare, with only a handful of cases being described in the world literature (Florman et al. 1973; Nahmias et al. 1983; Honig and Brown 1982; Monif et al. 1985; South et al. 1969).

The commonest source of neonatal HSV is said to be the mother's birth canal at the time of delivery (Nahmias et al. 1983). However, information about the risk of neonatal infection following delivery through the infected birth canal is scarce. Nahmias et al. (1971) found that 3 of 6 (50%) women with primary and 1 of 23 (4%) with recurrent genital herpes at the time of delivery gave birth to an infected infant. Further evidence that maternal infection is important comes from two studies that looked at risk factors in the mothers of babies with neonatal herpes. Whitley et al. (1980) found that 27 of 56 (48%) mothers had

Table 3.3. Neonatal herpes – sources of infection

Maternal	Transplacental – rare Birth canal; at delivery – common Primary > recurrent Post delivery (HSV infection of lips, fingers, breast)
Paternal	Post delivery (HSV infection of lips, fingers etc.)
Other family members, medical or nursing staff	Post delivery (HSV infection of lips, fingers etc.)

genital herpes during pregnancy or at delivery, and Sullivan-Bolyai et al. (1983) reported that 16 of 26 (62%) mothers had herpes at delivery. Infants born to mothers with primary HSV at the time of delivery appear to be at particular risk, probably because of the high viral titres, the almost invariable involvement of the cervix and the lack of neonatally acquired maternal antibodies (Nahmias et al. 1983).

The risk of delivery through an infected birth canal when the mother has recurrent herpes is undoubtedly lower. The duration of viral secretion is often short, the viral titres are usually low and the lesions are mostly on the external genitalia, in many circumstances well away from the introitus. A recent survey of paediatric and obstetric experts suggested that the risk of neonatal infection following birth through an infected birth canal in women with recurrent genital herpes was less than 5% (Binkin et al. 1984) and this view is supported by a recent survey wich showed that there were no cases of neonatal herpes occurring amongst 34 infants born to mothers with recurrent genital infections at the time of delivery (Prober et al. 1987).

The importance of passively acquired maternal antibodies has been the subject of considerable debate. Whitley et al. in 1980 studied 35 babies with neonatal herpes and found that 17 who had neutralising antibodies to HSV in a titre of 1 in 40 or greater had a similar outcome (severity of the illness and neurological sequelae) to 18 infants who had lower titres. In contrast, findings from a study by Yaeger et al. (1980) suggested that patients with milder disease had higher levels of antibody. Finally, a study conducted by Nahmias et al. in 1983 suggested that the presence of maternal antibodies prevented disseminated infections occurring but not localised ones. It is probably that passively acquired maternal antibody does offer some protection; however, this may only be partial, and the likelihood of neonatal herpes developing may depend not only on the antibody level at the time of delivery, but also on the amount of virus to which the infant is exposed.

The risk to the neonate from asymptomatic viral shedding in patients who do not have recurrent herpes has not been studied. It is likely, however, that the risk is similar to that seen in patients with recurrent genital herpes. It is possible that this group constitutes a greater risk to the neonate, as these patients may not have high levels of neutralising antibody and consequently viral titres may be relatively high. In addition, the lack of history and typical clinical features in the mother may delay diagnosis in the neonate.

Other documented sources of neonatal infection include mother to baby after delivery, father to baby (Douglas et al. 1983; Yaeger et al. 1983) and baby to baby (Francis et al. 1975; Linnemann et al. 1975). It has also been suggested that contact with other adults including hospital personnel may be implicated (Light 1979).

In conclusion, neonatal herpes is usually contracted from the mother via the birth canal. The greatest risk occurs when the mother has primary herpes, although a considerable number of infants will be infected by mothers who are unaware that they have herpes.

References

Anonymous (1981) Herpes simplex infections. Environmental Health Branch, Department of Health, Woden, Australia. Commun Dis Intell No 81/24

Anonymous (1983) Laboratory Centre for Disease Control. Laboratory reports of herpes viruses in Canada 1982. Can Dis Weekly Rep 9–12: 81–84

Adam E, Dreesman GE, Kaufman RH, Melnick JL (1980). Asymptomatic virus shedding after herpes genitalis. Am J Obstet Gynecol 137: 827–830

Baker DA, Plotkin SA (1979). Genital herpes simplex virus (HSV) isolation during pregnancy. Obstet. Gynecol 53 (suppl 3): 95–125

Barton IG, Kinghorn GR, Najem S, Al-Omar LS, Potter CW (1982). Incidence of herpes simplex virus type 1 and 2 isolated in patients with herpes genitalis in Sheffield. Br J Vener Dis 58:44–47

Becker TM, Blount JH, Guinan ME (1985). Genital herpes infections in private practice in the United States: 1966–1981. JAMA 253: 1601–1603

Bell DM, Holman RC, Pavan-Langston D (1982). Epidemiologic aspects of herpes simplex keratitis. Ann Ophthalmol 14: 421–422

Binkin NJ, Koplan JP, Cates W (1984). Preventing neonatal herpes – the value of weekly viral cultures in pregnant women with recurrent genital herpes. JAMA 251: 2816–2821

Black FL, Hierholzer WJ, Pinheiro F de P, et al. (1974) Evidence for persistence of infectious agents in isolated human populations. Am J Epidemiol 100: 230–250

Brown ZA, Kern ZA, Spruance SL, Overall JC (1979) Clinical and virologic course of herpes simplex genitalis. West J Med 130: 414–421

Bryson YJ, Dillon M, Lovett M, et al. (1983) Treatment of first episodes of genital herpes simplex virus infection with oral acyclovir. N Engl J Med 308: 916–921

Buddingh GJ, Schrum DR, Lancier JC, Guildry DJ (1953). Studies of the natural history of herpes simplex infections. Pediatrics 11: 595–610

Centers for Disease Control (1982) Genital herpes infections, United States, 1966–1979. MMWR 31, 137–139

Centifanto YM, Hildebrandt RJ, Held B, Kaufman HE (1971) Relationship of herpes simplex genital herpes and carcinoma of the cervix – population studies. Am J Obstet Gynecol 110: 690–692

Cesario TC, Poland JD, Wulff H, et al. (1969) Six years' experience with herpes simplex virus in a children's home. Am J Epidemiol 90: 416–422

Chang TW, Fiumara NJ, Weinstein L (1974) Genital herpes. Some clinical and laboratory observations. JAMA 229: 544–545

Corey L, Spear PG (1986) Infection with herpes simplex virus. (Second of two parts.) N Engl J Med 314: 749–757

Corey L, Nahmias AJ, Guinan ME, Benedetti JK, Critchlow CW, Holmes KK (1982) A trial of topical acyclovir in genital herpes virus infections. N Engl J Med 306: 1313–1319

Corey L, Adams HG, Brown ZA, Holmes KK (1983) Genital herpes simplex virus infections: clinical manifestations, course and complications. Ann Intern Med 98: 958–972

Darougar S, Wishart MS, Viswalingham ND (1985) Epidemiological and clinical features of primary herpes simplex virus ocular infection. Br J Ophthalmol 69: 2–6

Dawson CR (1984) Ocular herpes simplex virus infections. Clin Dermatol 2: 56–66

Deardourff SL, Deture FA, Drylee DM, Centifanto Y, Kaufman H (1974) Association between herpes hominis type 2 and the male genitourinary tract. J Urol 112: 126–127

Docherty JJ, Lohse MA, Delavia MF, et al. (1984) Incidence of herpes simplex virus types 1 and 2 in penile lesions of college men. J Med Virol 13: 163–170

Douglas JM, Corey L (1983) Fomites and herpes simplex viruses: a case of nonvenereal transmission? JAMA 250: 3093–3094

Douglas J, Schmidt O, Corey L (1983) Acquisition of neonatal HSV 1 infections from a paternal source contact. J Pediatr 103: 908–910

Douglas JM, Critchlow C, Benedetti J, et al. (1984) A double-blind study of oral acyclovir for suppression of recurrences of genital herpes simplex virus infection. N Engl J Med 310: 1551–1556

Dowdle WR, Nahmias AJ, Harwell RW, Pauls FP (1967) Association of antigenic type of herpes virus hominis with site of viral recovery. J Immunol 99: 974–980

Duncan MO, Bilgeri YR, Fehler HG, Ballard RC (1981) The diagnosis of sexually acquired genital ulcerations in black patients in Johannesburg. S Afr J Sex Trans Dis 1: 20–23

Embil JA, Stephens RG, Manual FR (1975) Prevalence of recurrent herpes labialis and aphthous ulcers among young adults on six continents. Can Med Assoc J 113: 627–630

Florman AL, Gershon AA, Blackett PR, Nahmias AJ (1973) Intrauterine infection with herpes simplex virus. Resultant congenital malformations. JAMA 225: 129–132

Francis DP, Herrman KL, MacMahon JR, Chavigny JR, Sanderlin KC (1975) Nosocomial and maternally acquired herpes virus hominus infections. A report of four cases in neonates. Am J Dis Child 129: 889–893

Guinan ME, MacCalman J, Kern ER, Overall JC, Spruance SL (1981) The course of untreated recurrent genital herpes simplex infection in 27 women. N Engl J Med 304: 759–763

Hanna L, Ostler HB, Keshishyan H (1976) Observed relations between herpetic lesions and antigenic types of herpesvirus hominis. Surv Ophthalmol 21, 110–114

Herrmann EC Jr (1967) Experiences in laboratory diagnosis of herpes simplex, varicella zoster and vaccinia virus infection in routine medical practice. Mayo Clin Proc 42: 744–753

Hindley DJ, Adler MW (1985) Genital herpes: an increasing problem? Genitourin Med 61: 56–58

Honig PJ, Brown D (1982) Congenital herpes simplex virus infection initially resembling epidermolysis bullosa. J Pediatr 101: 958–959

Jeansson S, Molin L (1974) On the occurrence of genital herpes simplex virus infection. Acta Dermatol 54: 479–485

Juretic M (1966) Natural history of herpetic infection. Helv Paediatr Acta 4: 356–368

Kalinyak JE, Fleagle G, Docherty JJ (1979) Incidence and distribution of herpes simplex virus 1 and 2 from genital lesions in college women. J Med Virol 1: 175–181

Kaufman HE (1978) Herpetic keratitis. Invest Opthalmol Vis Sci 17: 941–957

Kaufman RH, Gardner HL, Rawls WE, Dixon RE, Young RL (1973) Clinical features of herpes genitalis. Cancer Res 33: 1446–1451

Kawana T, Kawagoe K, Takizawa K, Chen JT, Kawaguchi T, Sakamoto S (1982) Clinical and virologic studies on female genital herpes. Obstet Gynecol 60: 456–461

Kinghorn GR, Turner EB, Barton IG, Potter CW, Burke CA, Fiddian AP (1983) Efficacy of topical acyclovir cream in first and recurrent episodes of genital herpes. Antiviral Res 3: 291–301

Krugman S (1952) Primary herpetic vulvovaginitis. Report of a case: Isolation and identification of herpes simplex virus. Pediatrics 9: 585–588

Lafferty WE, Coombs RW, Benedetti J, Critchlow C, Corey L (1987) Recurrences after oral and genital herpes simplex virus infection. Influence of site of infection and viral type. N Engl J Med 316: 1444–1449

Larson T, Bryson Y (1982) Fomites and herpes simplex virus: the toilet seat revisited. Abstract. Pediatr Res 16: 244

Leventon-Kriss S, Rannon L, Smetana Z, et al. (1983) Incidence in laboratory confirmed cases of herpes genitalis and neonatal herpes infections in Israel. Isr J Med Sci 19: 946–949

Light IJ (1979) Postnatal acquisition of HSV by the newborn infant: A review of the literature. Pediatrics 63: 480–482

Lindgren KM, Douglas RC Jr, Couch RB (1968) Significance of herpes virus hominis in respiratory secretion of man. N Engl J Med 278: 517–523

Linnemann CC Jr, Buckman TG, Light IJ, Ballard JL, Roizman B (1975) Transmission of herpes simplex type 1 in a nursery for the newborn. Identification of viral isolates by DNA "fingerprinting". Lancet i: 964–966

Luby JP, Gnann JW Jr, Alexander WJ, et al. (1984) A collaborative study of patient-initiated treatment of recurrent genital herpes with topical acyclovir or placebo. J Infect Dis: 150: 1–6

Manzella JP, McConville JH, Valenti W, Menegus MA, Swierkosz EM, Arens M (1984) An outbreak of herpes simplex virus type 1 gingivostomatitis in a dental hygiene practice. JAMA 252: 2019–2022

McCaughtry ML, Fleagle GS, Docherty JJ (1982) Inapparent genital herpes simplex virus infection in college women. J Med Virol 10: 283–290

Meheus A, Van Dyck E, Ursi JP, Ballard RC, Piot P (1983) Aetiology of genital ulcerations in Swaziland. Sex Trans Dis 10: 33–35

Mertz GJ, Critchlow CW, Benedetti J, et al. (1984) Double-blind placebo-controlled trial of oral acyclovir in first episode genital herpes simplex virus infection. JAMA 252: 1147–1151

Mertz GJ, Schmidt O, Jourden JL, et al. (1985) Frequency of acquisition of first episode genital infection with herpes simplex virus from symptomatic and asymptomatic source contacts. Sex Trans Dis 12: 33–39

Mindel A, Sutherland S (1983) Genital herpes – the disease and its treatment including intravenous acyclovir. J Antimicrob Chemother 12 [suppl B]: 51–59

Mindel A, Weller IVD, Faherty A, Sutherland S, Fiddian AP, Adler MW (1986) Acyclovir in first attacks of genital herpes and prevention of recurrences. Genitourin Med 62: 28–32

Mindel A, Kinghorn G, Allason-Jones E, et al. (1987) Treatment of first-attack genital herpes, Acyclovir versus inosine pranobex. Lancet i: 1171–1173

Mindel A, Coker DM, Faherty A, Williams P (1988) Recurrent genital herpes: clinical and virological features in men and women. Genitourin Med 64: 103–106

Monif GRG, Kellner KR, Donnelly WH (1985) Congenital herpes simplex type II infection. Am J Obstet Gynecol 152: 1000–1002

Montefiore D, Sogbetun AO, Anong CN (1980) Herpesvirus hominis type 2 infection in Ibadan. Problem of non-venereal transmission. Br J Vener Dis 56: 49–53

Nahmias AJ, Dowdle WR, Naib ZM, et al. (1968) Genital infection with herpesvirus hominis type 1 and 2 in children. Pediatrics 42: 659–666

Nahmias AJ, Dowdle WR, Naib ZM, Josey WE, McClone D, Domesick G (1969) Genital infection with type 2 herpes virus hominis. Br J Vener Dis 45: 294–298

Nahmias AJ, Josey WE, Naib ZM, Luce CF, Duffrey C (1970) Antibodies to herpesvirus hominis type 1 and 2 in humans. 1. Patients with genital herpetic infections. Am J Epidemiol 91: 539–546

Nahmias AJ, Josey WE, Naib ZM, Freeman MG, Fernandez RJ, Wheeler JH (1971) Perinatal risk associated with maternal genital herpes simplex virus infection. Am J Obstet Gynecol 110: 825–837

Nahmias AJ, Keyserling HH, Kerrick G (1983) Herpes simplex. In: Remington JS, Klein JO (eds) Infectious diseases of the fetus and new born infant. W B Saunders Philadelphia pp 156–190

Nerurkar LS, West F, May M, Madden DL, Sever JL (1983) Survival of herpes simplex virus in water specimens collected from hot tubs in spa facilities and on plastic surfaces. JAMA 250: 3081–3083

Nsanze H, Fast M, D'Costa LJ, Tukei P, Curran J, Ronald AR (1981) Genital ulcers in Kenya: a clinical and laboratory study. Br J Vener Dis 57: 378–381

Oh JO, Kimura SJ, Ostler HB (1975) Acute ocular infection by type 2 herpes simplex virus in adults. Arch Ophthalmol 93: 1123–1127

Overall JC Jr (1984) Dermatologic viral diseases. In: Galasso GJ, Merigan TC, Buchanan RA (eds) Antiviral agents and viral diseases of man, 2nd edn. Raven Press, New York. pp 247–312

Patterson A, Jones BR (1967) The management of ocular herpes. Trans Ophthalmol Soc UK 87: 59–84

Pavan-Langston D (1984) Ocular viral diseases. In: Galasso G, Merigan TC, Buchanan RA (eds) Antiviral agents and viral diseases of man, 2nd edn. Raven Press, New York, pp 207–245

Peutherer JF, Smith IW, Robertson OHH (1982) Genital infections with herpes simplex virus type 1. J Infect 4: 33–35

Prober CG, Sullender WM, Yasukawa LL, Au DS, Yeager AS, Arvin AM (1987) Low risk of herpes simplex virus infection in neonates exposed to the virus at the time of vaginal delivery with recurrent genital herpes simplex virus infection. N Engl J Med 316: 240–244

Rattray MC, Corey L, Reeves WC, Vontver LA, Holmes KK (1978) Recurrent genital herpes among women: symptomatic v. asymptomatic viral shedding. Br J Vener Dis 54: 262–265

Rawls WE, Tompkins WAF, Melnick JL (1969) The association of herpes virus type 2 and carcinoma of the uterine cervix. Am J Epidemiol 89: 547–554

Rawls WE, Gardner HL, Flanders RW, Lowry SP, Kaufman RH, Melnick JL (1971) Genital herpes in two social groups. Am J Obstet Gynecol 110: 682–689

Reeves WC, Corey L, Adams HG, Vontver LA, Holmes KK (1981) Risk of recurrence after first episode of genital herpes. Relation to HSV type and antibody response. N Engl J Med 305: 315–319

Scott TFM, Correll L, Blank H, et al. (1952) Some comments on herpetic infections in children with special emphasis on unusual manifestations. J Pediatr 41: 835–843

Seth P, Sundaram KR, Samantoray JC, et al. (1981) Seroepidemiologic study of herpes simplex virus type 1 and 2 in Delhi. Indian J Med Res 73: 475–483

Ship II, Brightman UJ, Laster LL (1967) The patient with recurrent apthous ulcers and the patient with recurrent herpes labialis. A study of two population samples. J Am Dent Assoc 75: 645–654

Shuster JJ, Kaufman HE, Nesburn AB (1981) Statistical analysis of the rate of recurrence of herpesvirus ocular epithelial diseases. Am J Ophthalmol 91: 328–331

Sogbetun AO, Montefiore P, Anong CN (1979) Herpesvirus hominis antibodies among children and young adults in Ibadan. Br J Vener Dis 55: 44–47

South MA, Tompkins WAF, Morris CR, Rawls WE (1969) Congenital malformation of the central nervous system associated with genital (type 2) herpesvirus. J Pediatr 75: 13–18

Sullivan-Bolyai J, Hull HF, Wilson C, Corey L (1983) Neonatal herpes simplex virus infection in King County, Washington. Increasing incidence and epidemiologic correlates. JAMA 250: 3059–3062

Tardieu JC, Friedel J (1983) Incidence of herpes simplex virus type 1 and 2 in herpes genitalis in Strasbourg, France. Br J Vener Dis 59: 138

Taylor DN, Duangmani C, Suvongse C, et al. (1984) The role of *Haemophilus ducreyi* in penile ulcers in Bangkok, Thailand. Sex Trans Dis 11: 148–151

Thin RN. Nabarro JM, Davidson Parker J, Fiddian AP (1983) Topical acyclovir in the treatment of initial genital herpes. Br J Vener Dis 59: 116–119

Tobias MI, Hermon YE (1983) Changing patterns of genital herpes. N Z Med J 96: 684–686

Turner R, Shehab Z, Osborne R, et al. (1982) Shedding and survival of herpes simplex virus from "fever blisters". Pediatrics 70: 547–549

Vesterinen E, Purola E, Saksela E, Leinikki P (1979) Clinical and virological findings in patients with cytologically diagnosed gynaecologic herpes simplex infections. Acta Cytol (Baltimore) 21: 199–205

Whitley RJ, Soong S-J, Dolin R, et al. (1977) Adenoarabinoside therapy of biopsy-proved herpes simplex virus encephalitis. National Institute of Allergy and Infectious Diseases Collaborative Antiviral Study. N Engl J Med 297: 289–294

Whitley RJ, Nahmias AJ, Visintine AM, Fleming CL, Alford CA (1980) The natural history of herpes simplex virus of mother and newborn. Pediatrics 66: 489–494

Whitley RJ, Soong S-J, Linneman C, Liu C, Pazin G, Alford CA (1982) Herpes simplex encephalitis. JAMA 247: 317–320

Willmott FE, Mair HJ (1978) Genital herpes virus infection in women attending a venereal disease clinic. Br J Vener Dis 54: 341–343

Yaeger AS, Arvin AM, Urbani LJ (1980) Relationship of antibody to outcome in neonatal herpes simplex virus infections. Infect Immun 29: 532–558

Yaeger AS, Ashley RL, Corey L (1983) Transmission of herpes simplex from father to neonate. J Paediatr 103: 905–907

Young SK, Rowe NH, Buchanan RA (1976) A clinical study for the control of facial mucocutaneous herpes virus infections. In: Characterisation of natural history in a professional school population. Oral Surg 41: 498–507

Chapter 4

Clinical Features: Locally Defined Sites

Disease of the Lips and Oral Cavity

Primary Infections

Acute gingivostomatitis is the commonest clinical manifestation of primary infection with HSV in children (Dodd et al. 1938; Sheridan and Herrman 1971). Many children exposed to the virus, however, develop only trivial symptoms or remain asymptomatic (Overall 1984). In the minority who do have symptomatic infections, the presenting symptoms include a sore throat, inability to eat, irritability, malaise, fever, myalgias and headache. In young infants, the predominant symptoms are fever, listlessness and an unwillingness to eat or drink, whereas older children or young adults complain of a sore throat (Dodd et al. 1938; Sheridan and Herrman 1971; Hale et al. 1963; Young et al. 1976; Buddingh et al. 1953; Evans and Dick 1964).

Lesions may involve the inner aspects of the lips, the buccal mucosa, gums, tongue, tonsils, pharynx and the hard and soft palate (Fig. 4.1) (Dodd et al. 1938). On examination, the patient is often febrile and the cervical lymph nodes are enlarged and tender. Lesions commence as painful vesicles and within a day or two these burst to leave ulcers. The ulcers are shallow and often have a yellow exudative base and an erythematous halo. By the time the patient presents to the physician there are usually extensive areas of ulceration and exudation. The lips may be swollen and the lesions may bleed when touched. Occasionally, especially in children, the disease may be severe enough to prevent eating or drinking and the child may be severely dehydrated (Dodd et al. 1938; Hale et al. 1963).

In young adults the disease may present as a pharyngitis with exudative ulcerative lesions on the pharynx, tonsils and buccal mucosa (Fig. 4.1). Some of these infections are probably contracted through oral–genital sexual contact (Sheridan and Herrman 1971; Silverman and Beumer 1973; Glenzen et al. 1975). The fever and local pain usually settle within 2 to 7 days, although complete healing takes anything from 1 to 4 weeks (Overall 1984). The reason

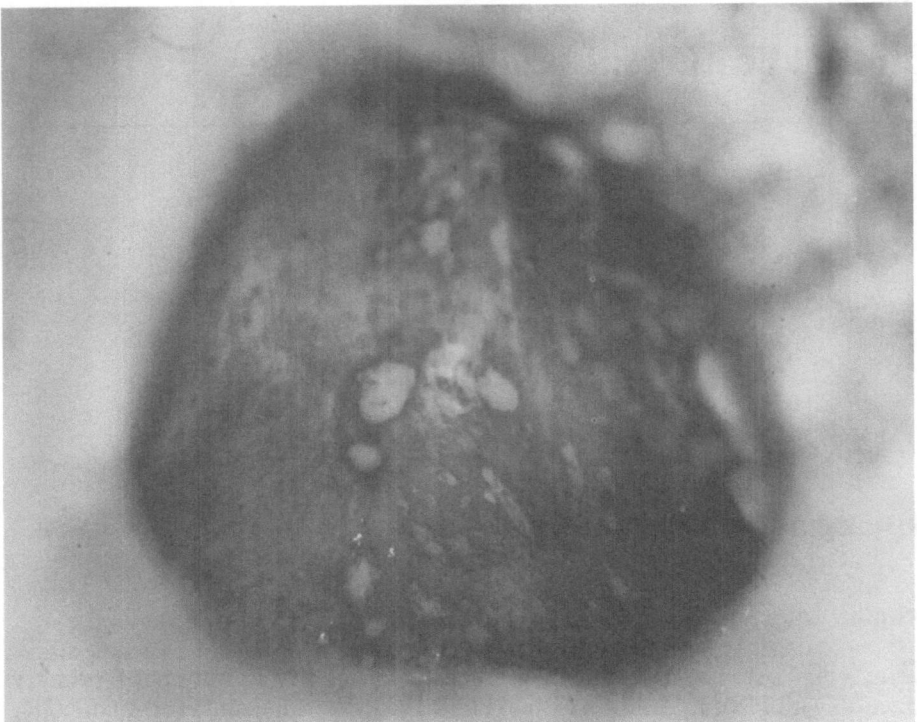

Fig. 4.1. Primary herpetic stomatitis: ulcers on the hard and soft palate.

for the prolonged time to healing in some patients is the observation that new lesions may occur on the tongue, cheek and lips in the second week of the illness in patients with a severe infection. Viral excretion may continue for up to 4 weeks (Buddingh et al. 1953).

The clinical diagnosis of acute gingivostomatitis usually poses no problems. Where the illness is confined to the buccal mucosa or the palate the possibility of coxsackie A, B and echo viruses causing the clinical entity herpangina need to be considered. Herpangina is usually less severe than primary herpetic gingivo-stomatitis, with the illness lasting only a few days. Where the disease presents with a pharyngitis, a variety of different conditions will need to be considered in the differential diagnosis. These include infectious mononucleosis, adenovirus infection, streptococcal sore throat, diphtheria, Vincent's angina and the possibility of non-infectious causes such as the Stevens–Johnson syndrome.

Recurrent Oral Herpes

The major differences between primary infection of the mouth and recurrent disease are summarised in Table 4.1. Cold sores (fever blisters or herpes labialis) are the commonest clinical manifestation of recurrent infection (Fig. 4.2) with herpes simplex. Spruance et al. (1977) have estimated that 65% to 85% of

Table 4.1. Differences between primary and recurrent oral herpes

	Primary	Recurrent
Site	Buccal mucosa, gums, tonsils, pharynx, palate.	Lips
No. of lesions	Multiple	80% single
Constitutional symptoms	Common	Rare
Duration of lesions	14–24 days	6–10 days
Duration of viral shedding	6–16 days	2–4 days
Viral titres	High	Low
Prodromal symptoms	No	Yes

patients with herpes labialis have prodromal or warning symptoms. These usually consist of pain, tingling or itching in the site of the subsequent lesions. The prodrome is followed within a few hours by small erythematous papules which rapidly progress to intradermal vesicles on the vermilion border of the lips or the adjacent facial skin (Fig. 4.2). Eighty per cent of patients have only a single lesion and only 5% have more than two lesions (Young et al. 1976; Spruance et al. 1977). Most vesicles are replaced in 24 to 48 h by ulcers, which rapidly dry out and form a scab (Spruance et al. 1977).

The illness lasts anything from 6 to 10 days, with pain usually only present for the first 24 to 36 h. Constitutional symptoms and lymphadenopathy are only

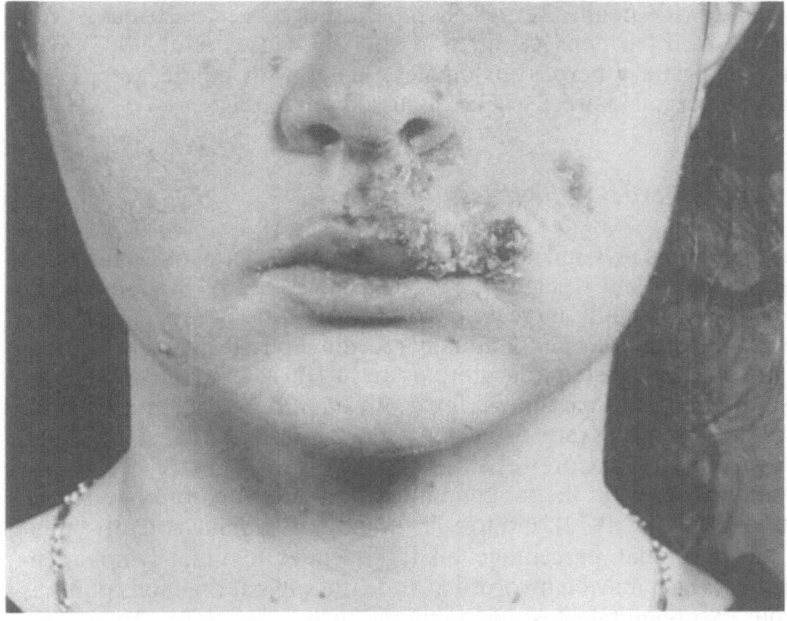

Fig. 4.2. Recurrent labial herpes (cold sores). Crusted lesions on the upper lip and nose.

rarely found (Oxman 1981; Young et al. 1976; Spruance et al. 1977; Juel-Jensen and MacCullum 1972). Virus may be isolated from the lesions, particularly during the papular and vesicular stages; thereafter viral excretion rapidly decreases (Overall 1984).

Occasionally patients with recurrent orolabial herpes have lesions in the oral cavity, either in the absence of lesions on the lips, or in conjunction with them (Douglas and Couch 1970). Such lesions may occur anywhere within the oral cavity, although the commonest site is the hard palate (Weathers and Griffin 1970). Virus may be isolated from such lesions and also from the oral cavity in the absence of obvious herpetic sores. Such asymptomatic infections are an important source of transmission (Spruance 1984).

Disease of the Genitalia and Adjacent Area

Primary Genital Herpes

The first attack of genital herpes is often characterised by extensive genital and perigenital ulceration (often lasting several weeks), severe local and systemic symptoms and a prolonged duration of virus excretion (Corey et al. 1983). Patients with clinical or serological evidence of previous HSV infection tend to have a milder first attack than those having a "true primary" infection. Both HSV 1 and 2 can cause first-attack genital herpes and the infections are clinically indistinguishable (Corey 1985). First-attack genital herpes is often more severe in females and in homosexual males with anal or perianal herpes than in heterosexual males with penile herpes. Symptoms occur 2 to 20 days after exposure to an infected partner (Kaufman et al. 1973; Corey et al. 1983). The clinical features of primary herpes in females, males with penile herpes and those with anal and perianal herpes will be discussed separately.

First-Attack Genital Herpes in Females

The presenting symptoms in women include vulval pain, groin pain, dysuria and vaginal discharge (Davis and Keeney 1981; Kaufman et al. 1973; Corey et al. 1983). Local symptoms usually increase over the first 6 to 7 days, reaching a maximum around the tenth day and gradually receding over the second week of the illness (Corey 1985). Systemic symptoms occur in a large percentage of patients. These include a flu-like illness, fever, myalgia, headache and abdominal pain. Systemic symptoms are usually of shorter duration than the local symptoms (Brown et al. 1979; Corey et al. 1983).

Lesions commonly occur on the labia minora and majora, clitoris, perineum and perianal area (Ng et al. 1970). Up to 80% of patients will have involvement of the cervix and a similar percentage bilateral tender inguinal lymphadenopathy. Other sites which may be involved include the vagina, the mons pubis as well as numerous extra-genital sites, including the rectum, pharynx, breast, lip, finger, eye, buttocks and groin (Corey et al. 1983). Corey et al (1983), studying

Fig. 4.3. Primary genital herpes: bilateral vulval ulceration.

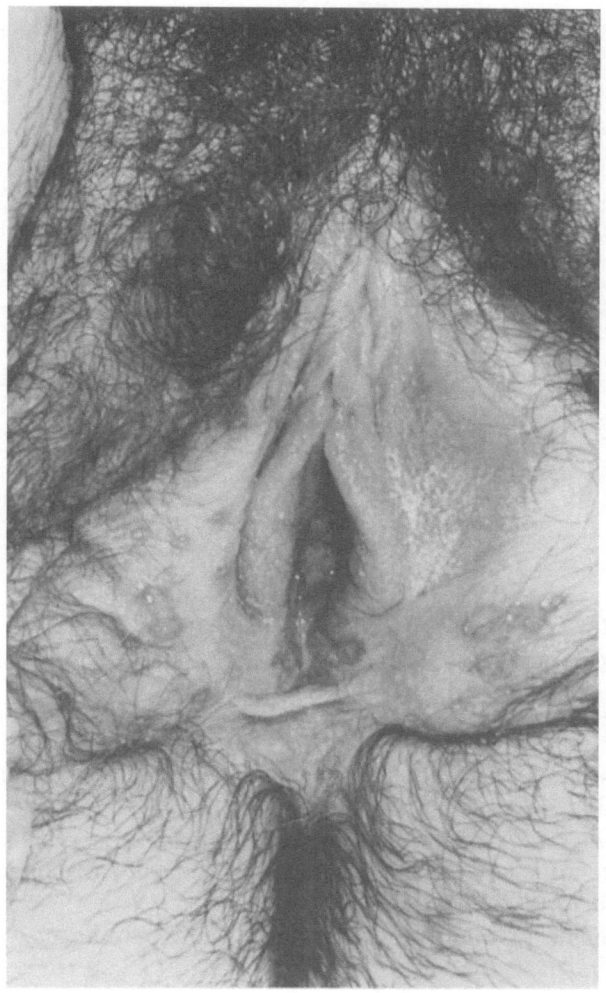

126 females with primary HSV 2 found that the mean duration of lesions was 19.7 days and that many continued to form new lesions up till the eighth day.

The lesions present as erythematous papules which vesiculate. The vesicles burst to leave ulcers with a erythematous halo and a greyish-white exudate in the base. Lesions on moist areas, for example labia minora, heal without crusting, whilst those on dry areas, for example mons or buttocks, heal with crusts or scabs (Poste et al. 1972; Brown et al. 1979). Lesions on the vulva are often widespread and diffuse, with areas of confluent ulceration (Figs. 4.3 and 4.4.) whereas those on extra-genital sites tend to be localised (Corey et al. 1983).

Several types of herpetic cervicitis have been described (Josey et al. 1966; Mindel and Codd 1984). They include:

Diffuse cervicitis, where the entire ectocervix is diffusely inflamed, oozing mucopus and bleeding easily at touch

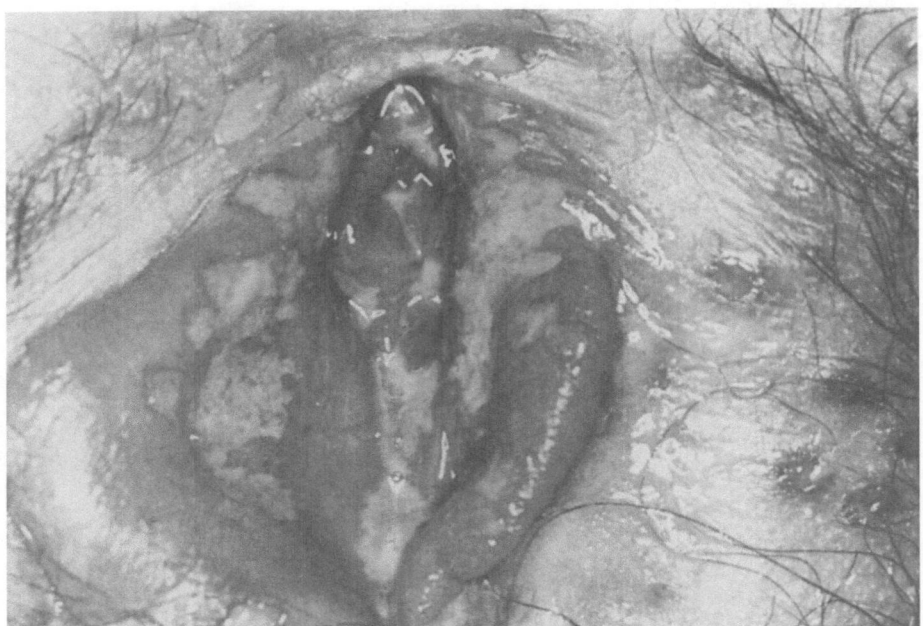

Fig. 4.4. Primary genital herpes: extensive vulval ulceration and swelling.

Multiple discreet ulcers, each with a greyish-white base and a erythematous halo (Fig. 4.5)

Necrotic cervicitis, where the entire ectocervix is heaped up, greyish and necrotic looking and is sometimes clinically indistinguishable from carcinoma of the cervix (Fig. 4.6)

Single or multiple deep ulcers; these may be up to a centimetre long and a similar depth

First-Attack Genital Herpes in Males

Primary herpes in males can occur on the penis, the perianal area and the anal canal. Penile herpes is a relatively mild infection, whereas perianal and anal herpes is often severe and prolonged.

Penile Herpes

The symptoms of penile herpes include pain in the genital area or groin, and dysuria if the lesions are near the urethra. Systemic symptoms are less common than in female patients (Corey et al. 1983).

Lesions can occur anywhere on the penis. The glans, coronal sulcus and foreskin are the commonest sites involved (Figs. 4.7 and 4.8). Eighty per cent of

Fig. 4.5. Primary genital herpes: discreet ulcers on the ectocervix.

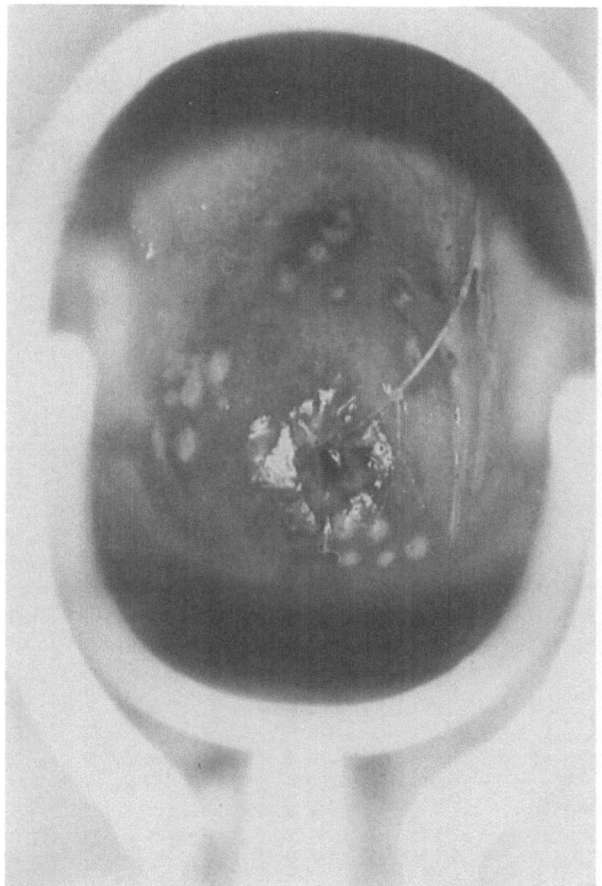

patients will have tender inguinal lymphadenopathy. Lesions progress through the same vesicular ulcerative crusting phases as in females. Lesions in moist sites (e.g. the glans in uncircumcised men) heal without crusting (Davis and Keeney 1981). As in female patients, extra-genital lesions are not uncommon (Crane and Lerner 1978; Glogau et al 1977; Sumers et al. 1980). The disease tends to be of shorter duration than in female patients, with a mean duration of lesions in men being 16.5 days compared with 19.7 in women (Corey et al. 1983).

Perianal and Anal Herpes

The first attack of anal herpes is usually a severe disease characterised by fever, inguinal lymphadenopathy, rectal discharge, pain and tenesmus. Goodell et al. (1983) studied the clinical features of 23 patients with herpes proctitis and compared them to 79 patients with non-herpetic proctitis. Significantly more patients with anal herpes had pain, tenesmus, pruritus, perianal lesions, inguinal lymphadenopathy and fever than those with non-HSV proctitis.

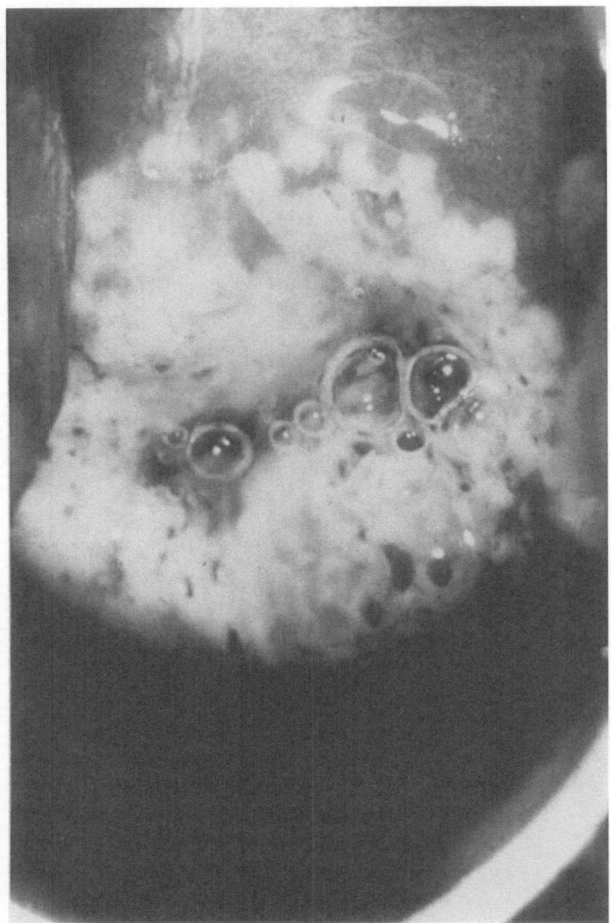

Fig. 4.6. Primary genital herpes: necrotic cervicitis.

The disease presents with an acute onset of pain, tenesmus and anal discharge, and the patient may notice perianal lesions. Examination reveals perianal vesicles, ulcers or scabs (Figs. 4.9 and 4.10). Proctoscopy is excruciatingly painful. The rectal mucosa is usually erythematous, covered in mucopus and friable, and the inflammation is almost always confined to the lower 10 cm of the rectum. The patient is often febrile and may complain of flu-like symptoms (Goodell et al. 1983; Corey 1985).

The illness often has a protracted course, with an average duration of symptoms being 17–21 days (Quinn 1981; Goodell et al. 1983; Samarasinghe et al. 1979) and some patients taking up to 4 weeks to heal (Waugh 1976).

Differential Diagnosis

The causes of genital ulceration are given in Table 4.2. Confirmation of the cause may depend on specific microbiological tests (see Chap. 7). The diagnosis

Table 4.2. Causes of genital ulceration

Infections
Genital herpes
  Primary
  Recurrent
Syphilis
  Primary chancre
  Secondary mucous patches
  Gummatous lesions
Candidosis
Trichomoniasis
Scabies
Chancroid
Lymphogranuloma venereum
Granuloma inguinale
Pyogenic infection
Folliculitis
Herpes zoster

Non-infective causes
Trauma
  Physical (e.g. sexual intercourse or masturbation)
  Chemical (e.g. antiseptics, caustic agents, etc.)
Reiter's syndrome (circinate balanitis)
Behçet's syndrome
Leukoplakia
Lichen sclerosis et atrophicus
Neoplasia (carcinoma penis/vulva)
Crohn's disease
Drug reactions (e.g. Stevens-Johnson syndrome)

of genital herpes should always be confirmed with a viral culture, and other sexually transmitted diseases excluded. Syphilis, although usually very different from herpes (the ulcer is usually single, indurated and painless and associated with painless lymphadenopathy – Fig. 4.11), should always be excluded. Behçet's syndrome, which may be confused with genital herpes because of the recurrent nature of the painful genital ulcers, may also need to be considered (Fig. 4.12).

Complications of First-Attack Genital Herpes

A number of complications have been described during or following the first attack of genital herpes. These include: dissemination to sites distant from the genitalia, meningitis, sacral radiculomyelopathy, urinary difficulties or retention, necrotising balanitis, synechia vulvae (fusion of the labia minora), urethral stricture, suppurative lymphangitis, salpingitis and secondary bacterial or fungal infection.

Extragenital Involvement (Figs. 4.13 and 4.14)

Extragenital involvement may occur from primary inoculation at sites such as fingers, pharynx or breasts, from haematogenous spread during the viraemic

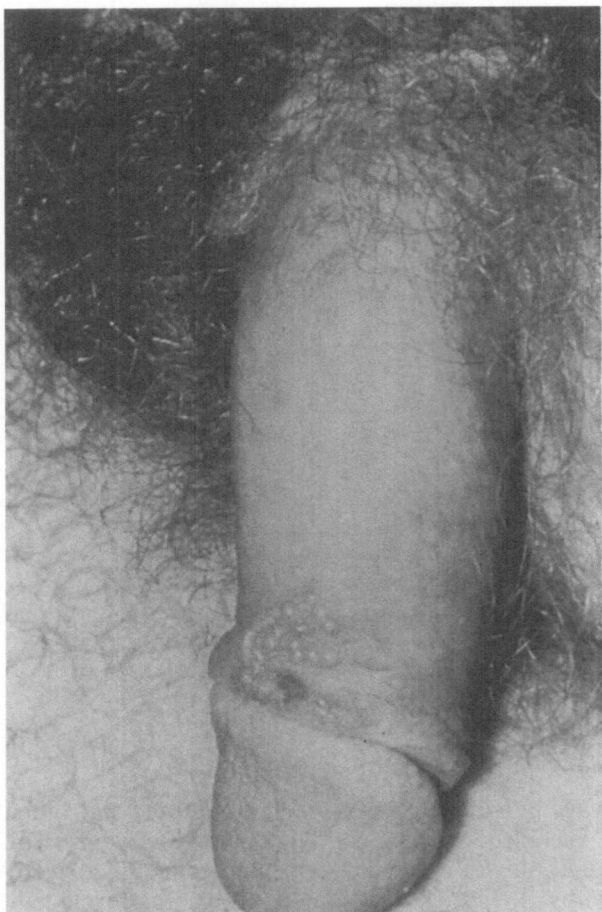

Fig. 4.7. Primary genital herpes: a crop of vesicles on the penis.

phase of the illness or from autoinoculation to any mucocutaneous site. The commonest sites of extragenital involvement are the fingers, and areas adjacent to the genitalia; suggesting that lesions arise from autoinoculation rather than viraemia (Corey et al. 1983).

Meningitis

Meningitis occurs in up to 36% of women and 13% of men with primary genital herpes (Corey et al. 1983). The clinical features include fever, headache, malaise, photophobia, neck stiffness and a positive Kernig's sign. The cerebro-spinal fluid shows a slight increase in levels of protein and lymphocytes. The condition, in common with most viral meningitides resolves within a few days without residual neurological sequelae (Sköldenberg et al. 1975; Meyer et al. 1960; Corey et al. 1983).

Fig. 4.8. Primary genital
herpes: diffuse ulceration of
the penis.

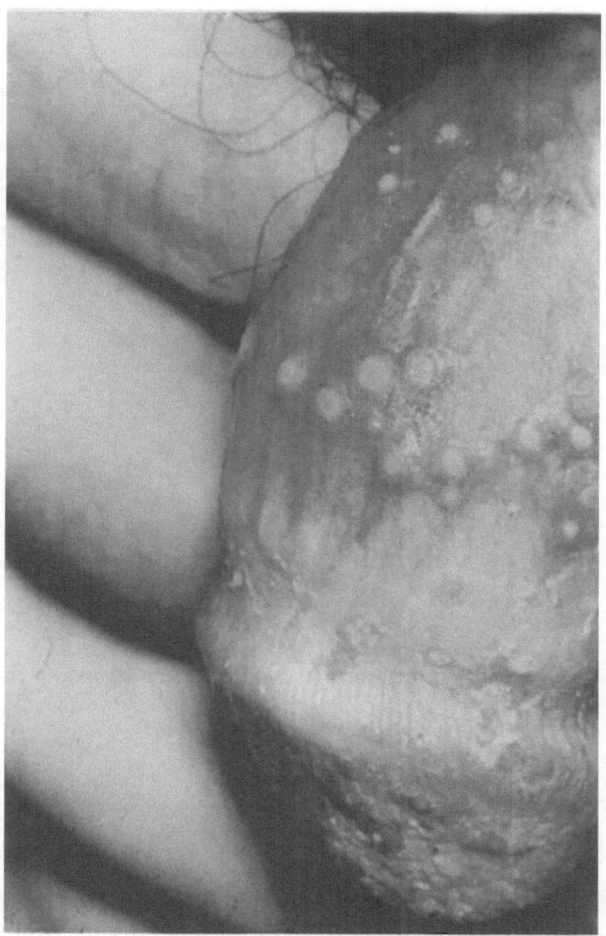

Sacral Radiculomyelopathy

Sacral radiculomyelopathy affecting the sensory and autonomic nerves occurs in
association with genital herpes (Klastersky et al. 1972; Caplan et al. 1977; Craig
and Nahmias 1973) and appears to be particularly common in homosexual men
with herpetic proctitis (Oates and Greenhouse 1978; Samarasinghe et al. 1979).
Signs and symptoms include hyperaesthesia or anaesthesia in the perineum,
thighs or buttocks, with decreased sensation over the sacral dermatomes, and
difficulty with urination and defaecation; there may also be poor rectal and
perianal sphincter tone, an enlarged bladder and an absent bulbocavernosus
reflex (Riehle and Williams 1979; Oates and Greenhouse 1978; Jacome and
Yanex 1980; Goldmeier et al. 1975; Samarasinghe et al. 1979). The pathogenesis
of this condition is unknown. The symptoms usually resolve in 2–3 weeks. The
condition usually occurs in association with severe overt herpetic proctitis,
although it has been described in patients with occult infection (Atia and Sonnex
1986).

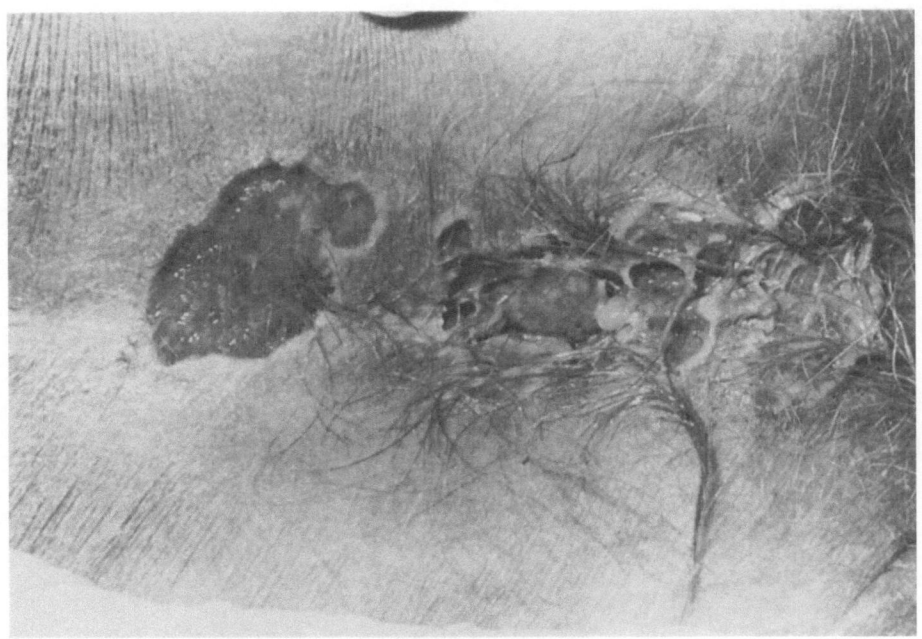

Fig. 4.9. Primary perianal herpes: extensive ulceration of the perianal skin.

Urinary Difficulties or Retention

Urinary problems occur commonly in patients with first-attack genital herpes, either because of severe pain associated with urethral or peri-urethral lesions (Nahmias and Roizman 1973) or because of the autonomic nervous system dysfunction described above. The problem is self-limiting although in severe cases catheterisation may be necessary (Corey et al. 1983).

Rare Complications

A number of rare complications have been attributed to herpes. Ortells (1921) described a man with a urethral stricture following repeated attacks of urethral herpes. Necrotising balanitis following herpes infection has been described by several workers (Powers et al. 1982; Peutherer et al. 1979). The condition appears to have a good prognosis. Other rare complications include a suppurative lymphangitis of the dorsum of the penis (Tottie 1942) and synechia vulvae (Brain 1956; DeMarco et al. 1987).

HSV may occasionally be isolated from the endometrium, Fallopian tubes and pouch of Douglas in women with pelvic inflammatory disease (Heinonen et al. 1985). The significance of these findings and the role of HSV in pelvic inflammatory disease has not been determined.

Fig. 4.10. Primary perianal herpes: area of localised ulceration.

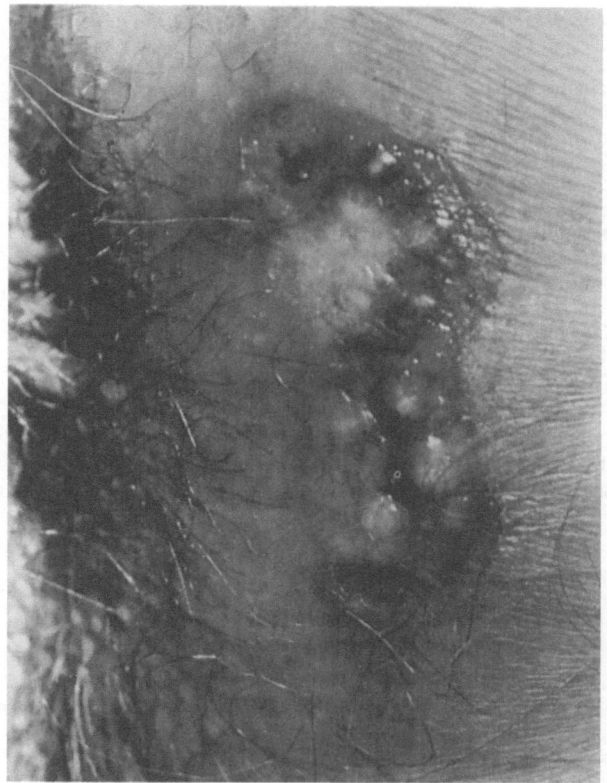

Recurrent Genital Infections

The major differences between first-attack and recurrent infection are shown in Table 4.3. Recurrences are usually of shorter duration and lesser severity and have a shorter duration of viral shedding than primary infections (Corey et al. 1983; Guinan et al. 1981). For example, Corey et al. (1983) found that the mean duration of lesions in women with recurrent infection was 9.3 days compared with 19.7 in primary infections.

Recurrent infections usually consist of a single or a small group of vesicles or ulcers at a single anatomical site (most often on the external genitals or buttocks; Fig. 4.15). Local symptoms are mild and systemic symptoms uncommon. The attacks last longer in men than in women (8.7 days versus 6.6. days), although more women have symptoms than do their male counterparts (Mindel et al. 1988).

For many patients the most troublesome aspects of recurrent genital herpes are, firstly, the frequency of recurrences and, secondly, the associated neuralgia-type pain. A considerable number of patients with HSV 2 will have frequent recurrences and it is not at all unusual to find patients with 12 or more recurrences per year (Mindel et al. 1988). Such patients may suffer profound emotional, sexual and psychological morbidity (see p. 61).

Table 4.3. Differences between primary and recurrent genital herpes

	First attack	Recurrences
Pain/dysuria	Severe	Absent–mild
No of lesions	Multiple	Few
Anatomical sites	Multiple	Usually single
Cervical involvement	80%–90%	<5%
Constitutional symptoms	Common	Rare
Prodromal symptoms	Unusual	Common
Duration of lesions	7–28 days	2–10 days
Duration of pain	5–20 days	1–7 days
Duration of viral shedding	5–25 days	1–10 days
Viral titres	High	Low
Radiculomyelopathy	≤50%	—
Meningitis	± 10%	—

Neuralgia-type pain radiating down the back of the thigh or in the buttocks, ankles or groin is a common accompaniment to recurrences. Sometimes the pain occurs at the same time as the recurrence and sometimes before, as part of the

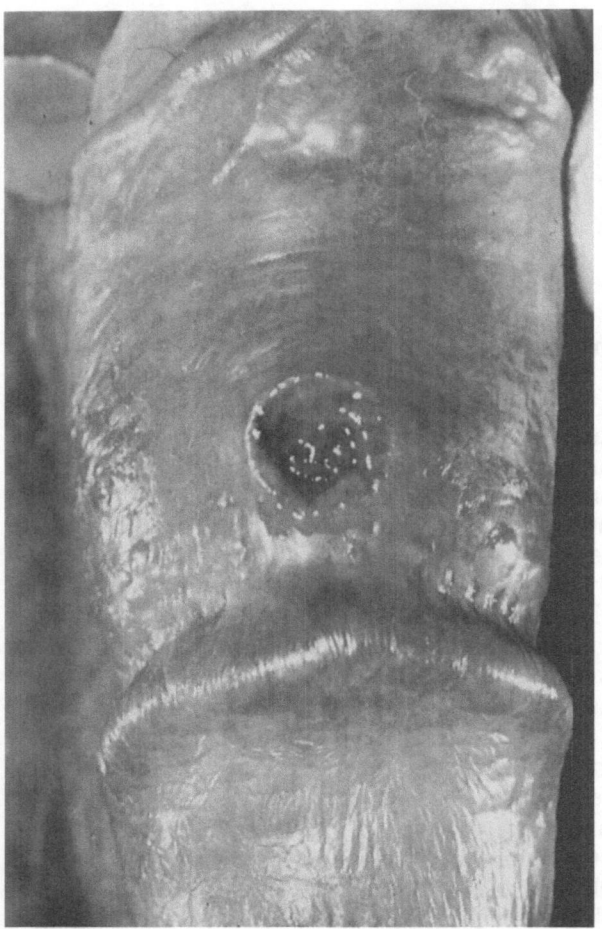

Fig. 4.11. Primary syphilitic chancre: single ulcer with heaped-up edges – usually painless.

Fig. 4.12. Behçet's syndrome: "punched out" ulcer on the scrotum.

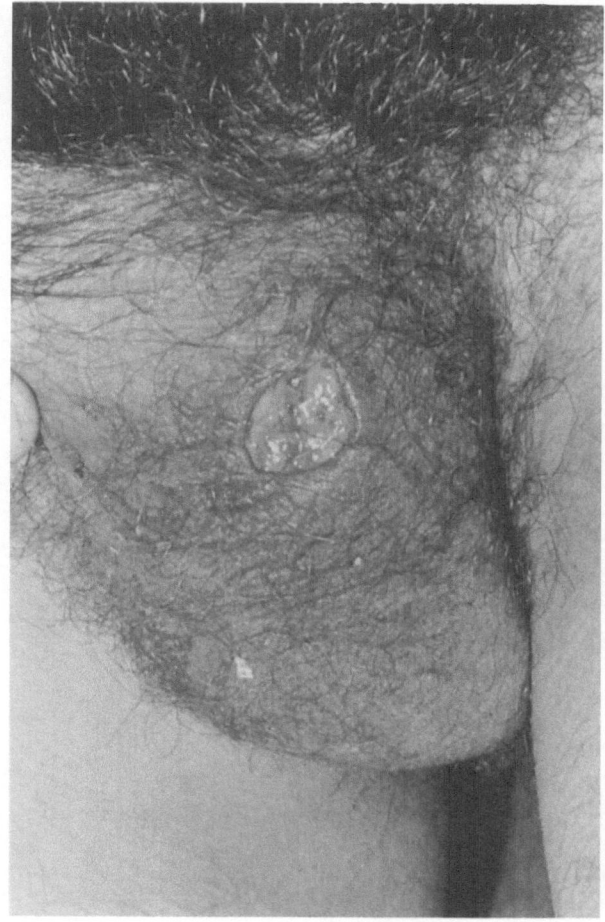

prodrome. The pain is often severe, may last for several days and occurs on occasion without any relationship to clinical recurrences. Other prodromal symptoms include hyperaethesias at the site where the lesions subsequently occur, malaise, fever and irritability.

Emotional and Psychological Morbidity Associated with Genital Herpes

Over recent years there has been considerable interest in the psychological issues concerned wth genital herpes. Several aspects have been identified, including the psychological and emotional reactions of the initial attack and its sequelae, alteration in sexual attitudes and behaviour, psychological and social adaption to having genital herpes and finally the relationship (if any) between stress and the frequency and severity of recurrences.

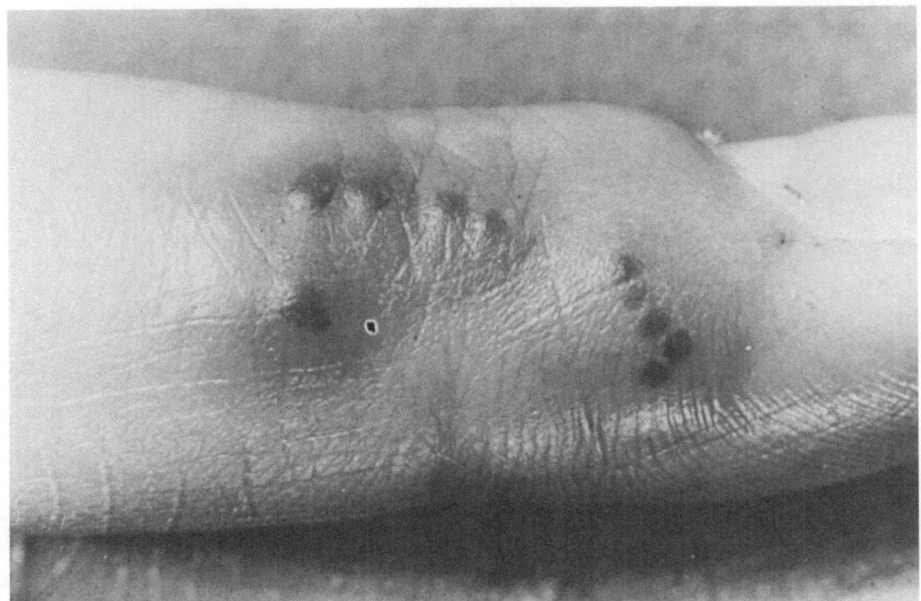

Fig. 4.13. Herpetic vesicles on the finger.

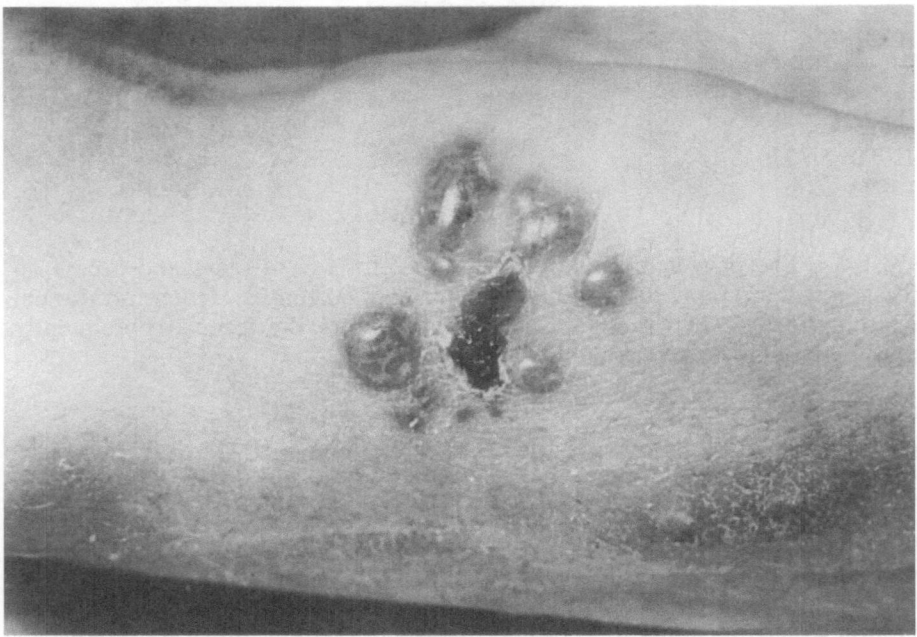

Fig. 4.14. Herpetic vesicles and crusts on the lateral aspect of the palm.

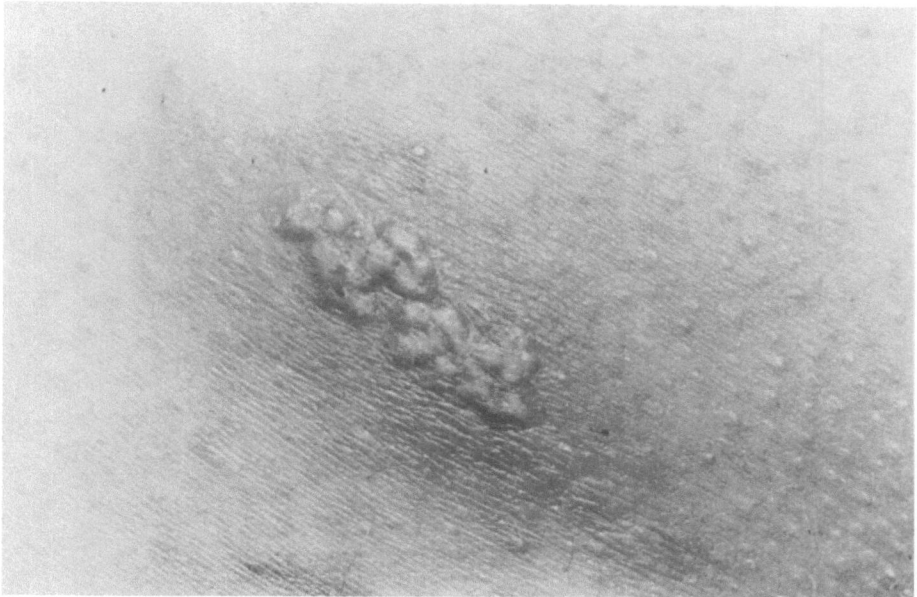

Fig. 4.15. Recurrent herpes: crop of vesicles on a buttock.

Psychological and Emotional reaction to the First Attack and its Sequelae

Anecdotal reports suggest that, following the diagnosis of initial genital herpes, many patients have a number of profound emotional reactions including depression, anger and hostility, helplessness and diminution of self-esteem (Lynch 1982; Bierman 1983; Marks and Patrick 1983; Sacher 1983).

The psychological reactions often occur sequentially (Fig. 4.16; A. Faherty, personal communication). At presentation, patients may be angry and disgusted. The anger is directed towards the person they feel has given them the illness and to some extent towards themselves for having contracted it. This feeling usually lasts only a few days. Disgust and a reduction in personal esteem are also common and these feelings tend to decrease or stop once the individual is feeling physically better and particularly when the obvious signs of illness (vesicles, ulcers and crusts) have healed.

The anger which is so common at the outset is replaced within a few days by feelings of bitterness and victimisation. "Why has this happened to me?" or "Will I ever be the same again?" are some of the typical responses. These emotions often last a long time and are interrelated with loss of self-esteem and sexual problems. These are discussed below.

Two particular problems often occur when the patient has recovered from the initial episode. One is denial and the other is anxiety about the future. In our experience, many patients refuse to acknowledge the fact that they ever had (or indeed continue to have) genital herpes. This may take the form of refusing to have a sexual relationship or, if they do indulge, not telling their partner that

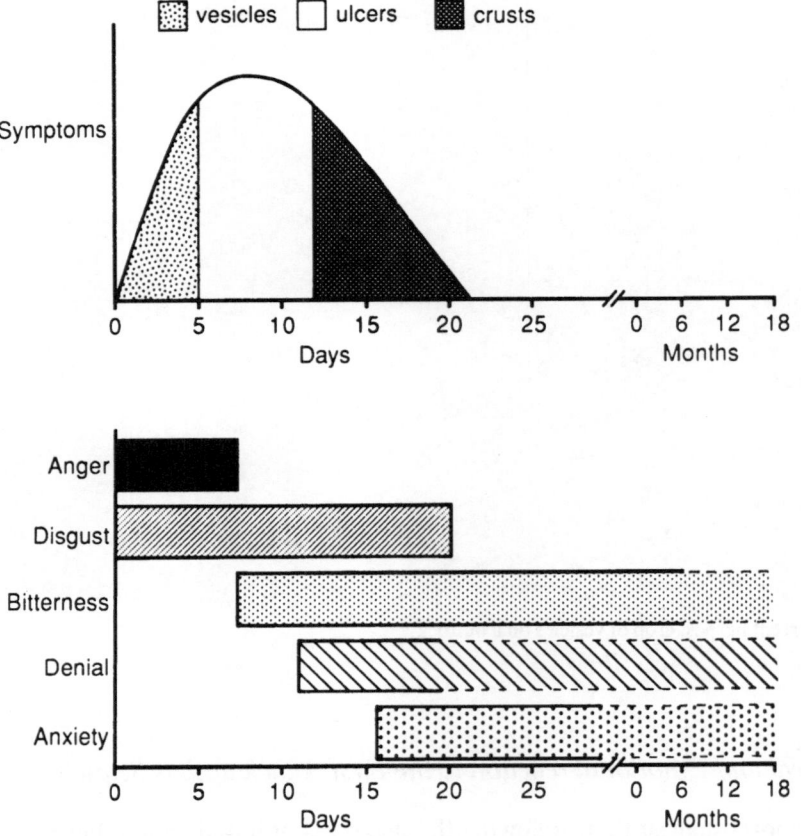

Fig. 4.16. Psychological morbidity (self-reported) associated with the first attack of genital herpes. Anger and disgust are early features, followed by bitterness, denial and anxiety. (By permission of Mrs A Faherty.)

they have the condition. This reaction is more common in women than in men (Mindel et al. 1988).

Anxiety about the future consequences of the illness is an important cause of morbidity. The anxiety is often multi-factorial, with patients concerned that they have a chronic "incurable" illness, that they may continue to have intermittent pain and discomfort for many years and that they will never be able to establish new sexual relationships. In women there is additional concern that the disease may be related to cervical carcinoma and that they may transmit the illness to any future children. Denial and/or anxiety may persist for many months or even years.

Alteration in Sexual Attitudes and Behaviour

Many patients may have considerable difficulty in talking to prospective (or existing) sexual partners about the illness. The difficulties include embarrassment in talking about sex and sexually transmitted diseases, and fear of rejection or censure (Blanks and Woddis 1983). Some individuals are so anxious about rejection and the effects that this may have on their desirability as sexual beings that they may choose not to disclose the illness to their partners or indeed avoid sex completely.

These responses may be self-perpetuating. Having been rejected once by a prospective sexual partner, some individuals will never "risk" the same thing happening again, whilst others, having "got away" with not telling, may feel that this is always the correct approach.

Patients who do have sexual relationships may also have problems. Many patients, particularly males, find that sex precipitates recurrences (Mindel et al. 1988) and in an attempt to reduce recurrences sexual activity may become less and less frequent, sometimes putting an enormous strain on the relationship. In some unfortunate individuals even masturbation brings on an attack, denying them even this form of sexual relief.

Psychological and Social Adaption to Genital herpes

A study by Manne and Sandler (1984) suggested that patients with poor psychological adjustment to genital herpes were those who indulged in wishful thinking, self-blame and negative thoughts. A positive factor was the level of social support. Whilst this study suggests that patients with recurrent genital herpes are not very different from patients with other "chronic" illnesses, the highly select nature of the study population (patients recruited from self-help groups and volunteers) suggests that these results should be interpreted with some caution. Whether the frequency or severity of recurrences is related to the degree of psychological morbidity is unknown.

Stress and Recurrences

It has long been believed that stress and herpes are related and there are several anecdotal reports and suggestions by physicians that this is indeed the case (Schneck 1947; Ullman 1947; Weichselbaum 1956; Hutfield 1968; Hamilton 1980; Blanks and Woddis 1983).

Several workers have studied the effects of stress on recurrent orolabial (Ship et al. 1967; Katcher et al. 1973; Luborsky et al. 1976) and genital herpes (Goldmeier and Johnson 1982; Goldmeier et al. 1986). The results of these studies have been either inconclusive or contradictory and interpretation has been further complicated by the definition and measurement of stress (numerous different questionnaires have been evaluated), the selection of patients (several studies have recruited highly select populations) and finally the timing of the questionnaires (patients studied at the time of the first attack or during recurrences are likely to have more emotional and psychlogical problems).

With so many other factors such as viral type, local trauma, menstruation, intercurrent infections and immune status known to be important in the pathogenesis of recurrences (see Chaps. 2 and 3) unravelling the importance of stress may prove to be very difficult.

Herpetic Hand Infection

Primary HSV infections of the hands occurs following exposure to the virus in susceptible individuals. Such infections may occur in health care workers following exposure to infected secretions (Stern et al. 1959; Louis and Silva 1979; Sehayik and Bassett 1982) or occasionally as a complication of primary genital or orolabial herpes either from finger-sucking or contact with infected genital secretions (Corey et al. 1983; Greaves et al. 1980; Feder and Long 1983; Crane and Lerner 1978; Glogau et al. 1977).

A recent study from Canada suggests that HSV infections may occur anywhere on the hand (Gill et al. 1988) and, although the finger is the commonest site involved (67%), the lateral or proximal nail fold is only rarely infected. The commonest sites are the digital pulp space and the lateral aspect of the fingers.

The disease presents with a sudden onset of pain, redness and swelling around the infected area. On examination, the patient is febrile and the infected site is erythematous and swollen, with several vesicular or even pustular lesions evident. The draining lymph nodes (including epitrochlear and axillary) are often swollen and tender, Spontaneous resolution usually occurs within 18–20 days (Corey and Spear 1986; Oxman 1981). Recurrences do occur but are less severe and of shorter duration.

Traumatic Herpes

Herpes infections on any skin site can occur when abraded skin is exposed to the virus. This type of infection has been described in laboratory workers (Nahmias and Roizman 1973), in wrestlers (herpes gladiatorum: Selling and Kibrick 1964; Wheeler and Cabaniss 1965; Porter and Baughman 1965) and following severe burns (see Chap. 5). Juel-Jensen and MacCullum (1972) described a primary HSV 1 infection in a baby with nappy rash. Herpetic whitlows may also be considered as a form of traumatic herpes. The lesions occur at the site of the trauma and are often accompanied by fever and regional lymphadenopathy. Recurrences may occur.

Eye Disease

Herpes simplex virus can cause a spectrum of eye diseases including conjunctivitis, keratitis, iridocyclitis, panuveitis, choroidoretinitis, cataracts and acute necrotising retinitis (Swyers et al 1967; Pavan-Langston and Brockhurst 1969; O'Connor 1976; Nahmias and Hagler 1972; Cogan et al. 1964; Cibis et al. 1978).

The commonest manifestation of HSV infection is keratitis, with or without involvement of the conjunctiva (Kaufman 1981). Uveitis is a rare complication of chronic stromal disease of the cornea (O'Connor 1976) and can on occasion lead to cataract formation (Nahmias and Hagler 1972). Choroidoretinitis and necrotising retinitis are seen only in neonates or in immunocompromised individuals (Nahmias and Hagler 1972; Cibis et al. 1978; Cogan et al. 1964).

Primary Infection

Primary herpetic eye disease occurs 3–9 days after exposure. The patient presents with a sudden onset of fever and blurring of vision, photophobia and a red eye. On examination, the preauricular lymph nodes are often enlarged and tender and the patient is febrile. Vesicles may be present on the eyelids and surrounding face. There is often chemosis and conjunctivitis (Pavan-Langston 1984; Binder 1977). Corneal lesions are initially diffuse; however, within 24 h multiple localised microdendrites or branching serpiginous lesions may be seen (Pavan-Langston 1984). In immunocompetent individuals the illness is self-limiting and corneal lesions usually heal without scarring.

Recurrent Ocular HSV Infection

Blepharitis and Conjunctivitis

Recurrent herpetic lesions of the eyelids have the same clinical features as lesions of the skin elsewhere, namely vesicles, ulcers and crusts (Fig. 4.17). Lesions occurring on the lid margin are often accompanied by a follicular (viral type) conjunctivitis (Dawson 1984). Conjunctivitis may occur in the absence of lid lesions. Corneal infection is common in association with conjunctival disease. Recurrent blepharoconjunctivitis may lead to blockage of the lacrimal drainage, with a marked increase in tear production (Coster and Welham 1979).

Recurrent Corneal Disease

Recurrent herpes infection of the cornea may cause a spectrum of diseases including one or more of the following: epithelial infectious ulcers, epithelial trophic ulcers or stromal disease (Patterson and Jones 1967; Pavan-Langston 1975).

The symptoms of recurrent epithelial ulcers include lacrimation, photophobia, irritation and sometimes blurred vision. Examination reveals typical branching dendritic ulcers (Fig. 4.18), which may be single or multiple, large or small. There may also be an associated conjunctivitis. Corneal sensation is often reduced, especially in patients with repeated recurrences. Patients with more severe disease may have stromal involvement (Pavan-Langston 1984).

In some cases the lesions progress to involve large areas of the epithelium. These defects are irregular and are often referred to as "geographical keratitis" (Pavan-Langston 1984; Dawson 1984). These ulcers are said to occur more commonly following the use of steroids. They are often long lasting and virus culture negative (Coleman et al. 1969).

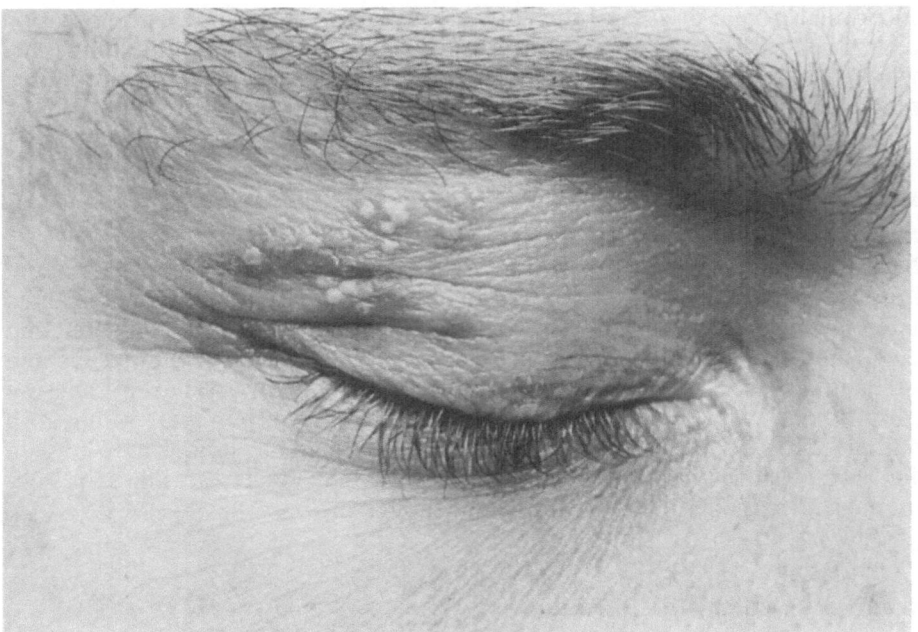

Fig. 4.17. Herpetic vesicles on the eyelid.

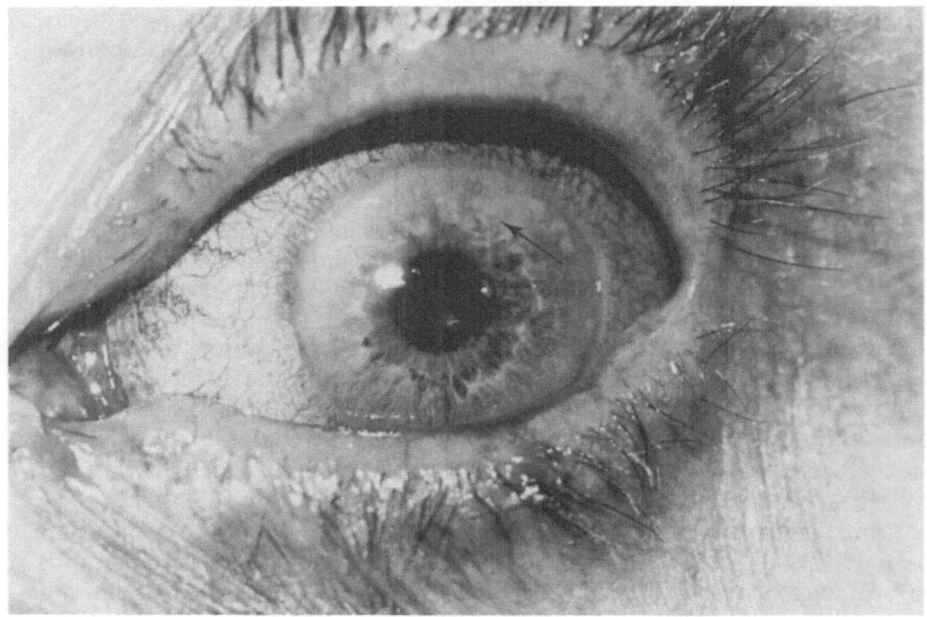

Fig. 4.18. Dendritic ulcers.

Ulcers near the limbus (the corneal/scleral junction) may be difficult to recognise, as typical dendritic or geographical ulcers may not occur (Thygeson 1971).

Epithelial Trophic Ulcers (Post-epithelial Ulceration)

Occasionally the cornea may ulcerate again a few days following recurrent epithelial ulceration. These ulcers are due to damage of the basement membrane during the infectious stage (Cavanagh 1975; Kaufman 1964).

Trophic ulcers are usually ovoid and need to be distinguished from infected geographical ulcers. Trophic ulcers have thickened, heaped-up borders whereas geographical ulcers are discrete, flat and may alter their configuration (Pavan-Langston 1984). Trophic ulcers may last for many weeks or even months and if left untreated may result in stromal melting and perforation (Cavanagh 1975).

Stromal Disease

Corneal stromal herpes (i.e. infection involving the connective tissue of the cornea) is more serious than epithelial infection, as it often results in permanent disability. Various clinical categories of stromal disease have been described. These include disciform oedema and various forms of necrotising stromal disease. Disciform oedema is characterised in its earliest phases by disc-shaped stromal oedema. The oedema leads to blurring of vision and as the disease progresses vascular invasion and scarring often occur (Thygeson and Kimura 1957).

Necrotising stromal disease can present as interstial keratitis resulting in a cheesy-white infiltrate which can obscure vision if it involves the visual axis. This form of stromal disease often results in scarring despite treatment (Fig. 4.19; see also Dawson 1984). Stromal disease is almost invariably accompanied by involvement of the uveal tract (Pavan-Langston 1984).

Herpetic Uveitis

HSV iridocyclitis or panvuveitis (O'Connor 1976; Pavan-Langston and Brockhurst 1969) is a frequent complication of corneal disease; although on occasion it may occur in the absence of obvious corneal involvement (Cavanagh 1975; Thygeson and Kimura 1957). The infection is characterised by a sudden onset of pain, photophobia and blurring of vision and redness of the eye (O'Connor 1976).

Examination reveals cells and flare and on occasion spontaneous haemorrhage or exudate (hypopyon) into the anterior chamber. Most adult infections are confined to the anterior chamber (Pavan-Langston and Brockhurst 1969).

In immunocompromised adults with HSV choroidoretinitis or encephalitis, and in neonatal herpes, the posterior uvea may be involved (Nahmias and Hagler 1972; see also Chap. 5).

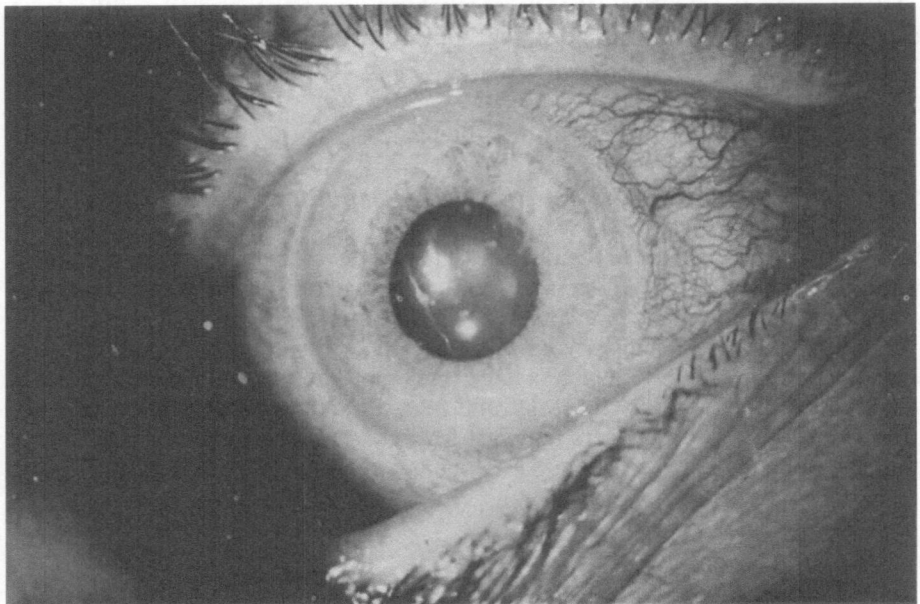

Fig. 4.19. Corneal scarring with marked limbal vasculitis.

Choroidoretinitis, Cataracts and Necrotising Retinitis

These rare manifestations of HSV ocular disease occur in immunocompromised patients or those with neonatal herpes (see Chap. 5).

References

Atia W, Sonnex C (1986) Retention of urine in occult anorectal herpes. Br Med J 292: 239

Bierman SM (1983) A possible psychoneurological basis for recurrent genital herpes simplex. West J Med 139: 547–552

Binder PS (1977) Herpes simplex keratitis. A review. Surv Ophthalmol 21: 313–331

Blanks S, Woddis C (1983) The herpes manual. Villiers Publications, London

Brain RT (1956) Clinical vagiaries of herpes virus. (Watson Smith Lecture.) Br Med J 1: 1061–1068

Brown ZA, Kern EA, Spruance SL, Overall JC (1979) Clinical and virologic course of herpes simplex genitalis. West J Med 130: 414–421

Buddingh GJ, Schrum SI, Lanier JC, Guidry DJ (1953) Studies of the natural history of herpes simplex infections. Paediatrics 11: 595–609

Caplan LRT, Kleeman FJ, Berg S (1977) Urinary retention probably secondary to herpes genitalis. N Engl J Med 297: 920–921

Cavanagh HD (1975) Management of inflammation associated with disciform keratitis and herpetic keratouveitis. In: Pavan-Langston D (ed) Ocular viral disease. Int Ophthalmol Clin 15: 67–88

Cibis GW, Flynn JT, David EB (1978) Herpes simplex retinitis. Arch Ophthalmol 96: 299–302

Cogan DG, Kowabana T, Young GF, Know DL (1964) Herpes simplex retinopathy in an infant. Arch Ophthalmol 72: 641–649

Coleman VR, Thygeson P, Dawson P, Jawetz EL (1969) Isolation of virus from herpetic keratitis. Influence of idoxuridine on isolation rate. Arch Ophthalmol 81: 22–24

Corey L (1985) Genital herpes. In: Holmes KK, Mårdh PA, Sparling PF, Wiesner PJ (eds) Sexually transmitted disease. McGraw Hill Book Company, New York, pp 449–474

Corey L, Spear PG (1986) Infections with herpes simplex viruses. (Second of two parts.) N Engl J Med 314: 749–757

Corey L, Adams HG, Brown ZA, Holmes KK (1983) Genital herpes simplex virus infections: Clinical manifestations, course, and complications. Intern Med 98: 958–972

Coster DJ, Welham RAN (1979) Herpetic canalicular obstruction. Br J Ophthalmol 63: 259–262

Craig C, Nahmias AJ (1973) Different patterns of neurologic involvement with herpes simplex virus types 1 and 2: isolation of herpes simplex virus type 2 from the buffy coat of 2 adults with meningitis. J Infect Dis 127: 365–372

Crane LR, Lerner AM (1978) Herpetic whitlow: a manifestation of primary infection with herpes simplex virus type 1 and 2. J Infect Dis 137: 855–856

Davis LG, Keeney RE (1981) Genital herpes simplex virus infection: clinical course and attempted therapy. Am J Hosp Pharmacol 38: 825–829

Dawson CR (1984) Ocular herpes simplex virus infections. Clin Dermatol 2: 56–66

DeMarco BJ, Crandell RS, Hreshchyshyn MM (1987) Labial agglutination secondary to a herpes simplex II infection. Am J Obstet Gynecol 157: 296–297

Dodd K, Johnston LM, Buddingh GJ (1938) Herpetic stomatitis. J Paediatr 12: 95–102

Douglas RG Jr, Couch RB (1970) A prospective study of chronic herpes simplex virus infection and recurrent herpes labialis in humans. J Immunol 104: 289–295

Evans AS, Dick EC (1964) Acute pharyngitis and tonsilitis in University of Wisconsin students. JAMA 190: 699–708

Feder HM, Long SS (1983) Herpetic whitlow: epidemiology, clinical characterisation, diagnosis and treatment. Am J Dis Child 137: 861–863

Gill MJ, Arlette J, Buchan K (1988) Herpes simplex virus infection of the hand. A profile of 79 cases. Am J Med 84: 89–93

Glenzen WP, Fernald GW, Lohr JA (1975) Acute respiratory disease of university students with special reference to the etiologic role of herpes virus in humans. Am J Epidemiol 101: 111–121

Glogau R, Hanna L, Jawetz E (1977) Herpetic whitlow as part of genital virus infection. J Infect Dis 136: 689–692

Goldmeier D, Johnson A (1982) Does psychiatric illness affect the recurrence of genital herpes? Br J Vener Dis 58: 819–828

Goldmeier D, Bateman JRM, Rodin P (1975) Urinary retention and intestinal obstruction associated with anorectal herpes simplex virus infection. Br Med J 1: 425–426

Goldmeier D, Johnson A, Jeffries D. et al. (1986) Psychological aspects of recurrences of genital herpes. J Psychomatic Res 30: 601–608

Goodell SE, Quinn TC, Mkrtichian E, Schuffler MD, Holmes KK, Corey L (1983) Herpes simplex virus proctitis in homosexual men: clinical sigmoidoscopic and histopathological features. N Engl J Med 308: 869–871

Greaves WL, Kaiser AB, Alford RH, Schaffner W (1980) The problem of herpetic whitlow among hospital personnel. Infect Control 1: 381–385

Guinan ME, MacCalman J, Kern ER, Overall JC, Spruance SL (1981) The course of untreated recurrent genital herpes simplex infection in 27 women. N Engl J Med 304: 759–763

Hale BD, Rentdorff RC, Walker LC, Roberts AN (1963) Epidemic herpetic stomatitis in an orphanage nursery. JAMA 183: 1068–1072

Hamilton R (1980) The herpes book. Houghton Mifflin, Boston.

Heinonen PK, Teisala K, Punnonen R, Miettinen A, Lehtinen M, Paavonen J (1985) Anatomic sites of upper genital tract infection. Obstet Gynecol 66: 384–390

Hutfield DC (1968) Herpes genitalis. Br J Vener Dis 44: 241–250

Jacome DF, Yanez GF (1980) Herpes genitalis and neurogenic bladder and bowel. J Urol 124: 752

Josey WE, Nahmias AJ, Naib ZM, Utley FM, McKenzie WJ, Coleman MT (1966) Genital herpes simplex virus infection in the female. Am J Obstet Gynecol 96: 493–501

Juel-Jensen BE, MacCullum FO (1972) Herpes simplex, varicella, and zoster: clinical manifestations and treatment. J P Lippincott Company, Philadelphia

Katcher AH, Brightman VJ, Luborsky L, Ship I (1973) Prediction of the incidence of recurrent herpes labialis and systemic illness from psychological measures. J Dent Res 52: 49–58

Kaufman HE (1964) Epithelial erosion syndrome: metaherpetic keratitis. Am J Ophthalmol 56: 984–987

Kaufman HE (1981) Local therapy of herpes simplex virus ocular infections. In: Nahmias AJ,

Dowdle WR, Schinazi RF (eds) The human herpesvirus. Elsevier, New York, pp 466–477

Kaufman RH, Gardner HL, Rawls WE, Dixon RE, Young RL (1973) Clinical features of herpes genitalis. Cancer Res 33: 1446–1451

Klastersky J, Cappel R, Snoeck JM, Flament J, Thirty L (1972) Ascending myelitis in association with herpes simplex virus. N Engl J Med 287: 182–184

Louis DS, Silva J (1979) Herpetic whitlow: herpetic infections of the digits. Am J Hand Surg 4: 90–93

Luborsky L, Mintz L, Brightman J, Katcher A (1976) Herpes simplex virus and moods: a longitudinal study. J Psychosomatic Res 20: 543–548

Lynch JM (1982) Helping patients through the recurring nightmare of herpes. Nursing 12: 52–57

Manne S, Sandler I (1984) Coping and adjustment to genital herpes. J Behav Med 7: 391–410

Marks LN, Patrick NH (1983) I think I may have herpes . . . What should I do? Occup Health Saf 52: 15–42

Meyer HM, Johnson RT, Crawford IP, Dascomb HE, Rogers NG (1960) Central nervous system syndromes of viral etiology: a study of 713 cases. Am J Med 29: 334–347

Mindel A, Codd MB (1984) Atypical herpes cervicitis: a case report. Eur J Sex Transm Dis 1: 201–202

Mindel A, Coker DM, Faherty A, Williams P (1988) Recurrent genital herpes: clinical and virological features in men and women. Genitourin Med 64: 103–106

Nahmias AJ, Hagler WS (1972) Ocular manifestations of herpes simplex in the newborn (neonatal ocular herpes). Int Ophthalmol Clin 12: 191–213

Nahmias AJ, Roizman B (1973) Infection with herpes simplex virus 1 and 2. (Third of three parts.) N Engl J Med 289: 781–789

Ng ABP, Reagan JW, Yen SSC (1970) Herpes genitalis clinical and cytopathologic experience with 256 patients. Obstet Gynecol 36: 645–651

Oates JK, Greenhouse PRDH (1978) Retention of urine in anogenital herpetic infection. Lancet i: 691–692

O'Connor GR (1976) Recurrent herpes simplex uveitis in humans. Surv Ophthalmol 21: 165–170

Ortells C (1921) Urethritis herpetica. Zentralbl Haut Geschlechskrankh 2: 122 (Abstract)

Overall JC Jr (1984) Dermatologic viral diseases In: Galasso GJ, Merigan TC, Buchanan RA (eds) Antiviral agents and viral diseases of man, 2nd edn. Raven Press, New York, pp 247–312

Oxman MN (1981) Herpes stomatitis. In: Braude AI, Davis CE, Fierer J (eds) Medical microbiology and infectious diseases. W B Saunders, Philadelphia, London, Toronto, pp 860–881

Patterson A, Jones BR (1967) The management of ocular herpes. Trans Ophthalmol Soc U K 87: 59–84

Pavan-Langston D (1975) Diagnosis and management of herpes simplex ocular infection. In: Pavan-Langston D (ed) Ocular viral disease. Int Ophthalmol Clin 15: 19–35

Pavan-Langston D (1984) Ocular viral disease. In: Galasso GJ, Merigan TC, Buchanan RA (eds) Antiviral agents and viral disease of man, 2nd ed. Raven Press, New York, pp 207–245

Pavan-Langston D, Brockhurst R (1969) Herpes simplex panuveitis. A clinical report. Arch Opthalmol 81: 783–787

Peutherer JF, Smith IW, Robertson DHH (1979) Necrotising balanitis due to a generalised primary infection with herpes simplex virus type 2. Br J Vener Dis 55: 48–51

Porter PS, Baughman RD (1965) Epidemiology of herpes simplex among wrestlers. JAMA 194: 998–1000

Poste G, Hawkings DF, Thomlinson J (1972) Herpes virus hominis infection of the female genital tract. Obstet Gynecol 40: 871–890

Powers RD, Rein MF, Hayden FG (1982) Necrotizing balanitis due to herpes simplex type 1. JAMA 248: 215–216

Quinn TC (1981) The etiology of anorectal infection in homosexual men. Am J Med: 71: 395–406

Riehle RA, Williams JJ (1979) Transient neuropathic bladder following herpes simplex genitalis. J Urol 122: 263–264

Sacher JB (1983) Coping and living with herpes. J Coll Health 31: 261–262

Samarasinghe PL, Oates JK, MacLenan IPB (1979) Herpetic proctitis and sacral radiculomyelopathy – a hazard for homosexual men. Br Med J 281: 365–366

Schneck JM (1947) The psychological component in a case of herpes simplex. Psychosomatic Med 9: 62–64

Sehayik RI, Bassett FH (1982) Herpes simplex infection involving the hand. Clin Orthop 166: 138–140

Selling B, Kibrick S (1964) An outbreak of herpes simplex among wrestlers (herpes gladiatorum). N Engl J Med 270: 979–982

Sheridan PJ, Herrman EC Jr (1971) Intraoral lesions of adults associated with herpes simplex virus. Oral Surg 32: 390–397

Ship II, Brightman VJ, Laster LL (1967) The patient with herpes labialis: a study of two population samples. J Am Dent Assoc 75: 645–654

Silverman S Jr, Beumer J III (1973) Primary herpetic gingivostomatitis of adult onset. Oral Surg 36: 496–503

Sköldenberg B, Jeansson S, Wolontis S (1975) Herpes simplex virus type 2 and acute aseptic meningitis: clinical features of cases with isolation of herpes simplex virus from cerebrospinal fluids. Scand J Infect Dis 7: 227–232

Spruance SL (1984) Pathogenesis of herpes simplex labialis: excretion of virus in the oral cavity. J Clin Microbiol 675–679

Spruance SL, Overall JC, Kern ER, Kreuger GC, Pliam V, Miller W (1977) The natural history of recurrent herpes simplex labialis. N Engl J Med 297: 69–75

Stern H, Elek SO, Millar OM, Anderson HF (1959) Herpetic whitlow. A form of cross-infection in hospitals. Lancet ii: 871–874

Sumers KD, Sugar J, Levine R (1980) Endogenous dissemination of genital herpes virus hominis type 2 of the eye. Br J Ophthalmol 64: 770–772

Swyers JS, Lausch RN, Kaufman HE (1967) Corneal hypersensitivity to herpes simplex. Br J Ophthalmol 51: 843–846

Thygeson P (1971) Marginal herpes simplex keratitis simulating catarrhal ulcer. Invest Ophthalmol 10: 1006

Thygeson P, Kimura S (1957) Deep forms of herpetic keratitis. Am J Ophthalmol 43: 109–113

Tottie M (1942) Herpes genitalis subsequente bubonulo. Acta Derm Venereol (Stockh) 23: 306–309

Ullman M (1947) Herpes simplex and second degree burns induced under hypnosis. Am J Psychiatry 103: 824–830

Waugh MA (1976) Anorectal herpesvirus hominis infection in men. J Am Vener Dis Assoc 31, 68–70

Weathers DR, Griffin JW (1970) Intraoral ulceration of recurrent herpes simplex and recurrent aphthae: two distinct clinical entities. J Am Dent Assoc 81: 81–88

Weichselbaum P (1956) Herpes recurrens – emotional factors. Psychosomatic Med 18: 81–83

Wheeler EC Jr, Cabaniss WH Jr (1965) Epidemic cutaneous herpes simplex in wrestlers (herpes gladiatorum) JAMA 194: 993–997

Young SK, Rowe NH, Buchanan RA (1976) A clinical study for the control of facial mucocutaneous herpes virus infection. 1. Characterization of natural history in a professional school population. Oral Surg 41: 498–507

Chapter 5

Clinical Features: Disseminated Infection

Introduction

Local or visceral dissemination of HSV infection can occur in a variety of clinical situations. These include immunocompromised patients, patients with severe infections, malnutrition or skin disorders and in neonates. In addition, dissemination may occur with pregnancy and occasionally in apparently normal individuals (Table 5.1).

Table 5.1. Conditions associated with disseminated HSV infection

1. Neonates
2. Immunosuppression
Congenital
Wiskott–Aldrich Syndrome
Acquired
Tumours: lymphomas, leukaemias, others
Immunosuppressive therapy
Acquired immune deficiency syndrome
Infections: measles, tuberculosis, whooping cough, pneumonia
Malnutrition
3. Skin disorders
Atopic eczema
Burns
Autosomal dominant ichthyosis vulgaris
Darier's disease
Familial benign pemphigus
Pemphigus foliaceus
Congenital ichthyosiform erythroderma
4. Pregnancy
5. Normal individuals

Perinatal Infection

The majority of perinatal infections occur at the time of, or soon after, delivery. Infection occurring via the transplacental route has been described in a handful of cases worldwide. The clinical features of these cases include central nervous system involvement, with intracranial calcification, microcephaly and profound mental retardation, eye involvement including choroidoretinitis, microphthalmia and retinal dysplasia, short digitis and recurrent cutaneous HSV infections (Florman et al. 1973; Nahmias et al. 1970, 1983a; Honig and Brown 1982; Monif et al. 1985; South et al. 1969).

Infection acquired at the time of delivery or postnatally (see Chap. 3) is recognised in the first week of life in 66% of cases; however, infection can occur up to 4 weeks after delivery (Sullivan-Bolyai et al. 1983; Stagno and Whitley 1985). The disease has been classified as disseminated, or localised (Table 5.2; see also Nahmias et al. 1983a; Alford 1984). Neonates with disseminated infection usually present within the first week; those with localised disease occur later, mostly at around the 11th day (Nahmias et al. 1983a). Approximately half the infants are born prematurely (Whitley et al. 1980a; Nahmias et al. 1983a).

Table 5.2. Clinical spectrum associated with neonatal herpes

Clinical features	% of cases
Disseminated without CNS involvement	22
Disseminated with CNS involvement	32
Localised CNS	29
Localised eye	4
Localised skin	12
Localised oral	1

Based on Nahmias et al. 1983a.
CNS, central nervous system.

Disseminated Infections

Disseminated HSV may be difficult to diagnose as the clinical features often resemble other severe neonatal diseases (Jenista 1984). The presentation is non-specific, with irritability, poor appetite and lethargy. Within 24 h the infant may develop fever, respiratory distress, seizures and hepatomegaly, with or without jaundice (Arvin et al. 1982; Nahmias et al. 1983a). A rash is often not visible at presentation but subsequently develops in up to 50% of cases (Alford 1984). This may be a typical vesicular or ulcerative herpetic rash; however, other types of skin involvement occur, including a generalised macular or petechial rash or areas of denuded skin (Nahmias et al. 1983a).

When the central nervous system (CNS) is involved, the clinical manifestations include irritability, seizures, bulging fontanelle, opisthotonos and long tract signs. The cerebrospinal fluid (CSF) shows a moderate elevation in the number of lymphocytes and very high protein levels (Nahmias et al. 1983a). The CSF may, however, be normal (Arvin et al. 1982). CNS involvement occurs in up to 50% of infants with disseminated infection, and is the cause of death, usually within 2 weeks of the presentation, in the majority. Those that survive have profound psychomotor retardation with or without microcephaly and choroidoretinitis (Nahmias et al. 1983a; Whitley et al. 1980a, b). When the CNS is not involved, the clinical picture and subsequent mortality are dominated by involvement of the lungs and the haematopoetic system. In these cases, respiratory failure or a bleeding diathesis (characterised by thrombocytopenia and disseminated intravascular coagulation) is the major cause of death (Whitley et al. 1980a).

Localised Disease

Localised CNS disease (i.e. infection of CNS with no visceral involvement but often involving the skin) occurs in up to 15% of cases (Nahmias et al. 1983a). This infection is clinically similar to the CNS disease seen in disseminated infection, except that it occurs later and has a lower mortality. Localised skin involvement occurs in up to 10% of cases. Lesions can occur anywhere on the body and are particularly common on the presenting parts at delivery (usually the scalp or buttocks). Skin lesions, whether localised or part of a disseminated infection usually commence as vesicles with an erythematous base; these rapidly ulcerate and heal by scabbing, over the following 10–14 days. The lesion can be single or multiple and may occur in crops (Nahmias et al. 1983a; Whitley et al. 1980a, b) (Figs. 5.1, 5.2 and 5.3). There is no associated mortality with localised skin infections. Various atypical rashes have been described. These include

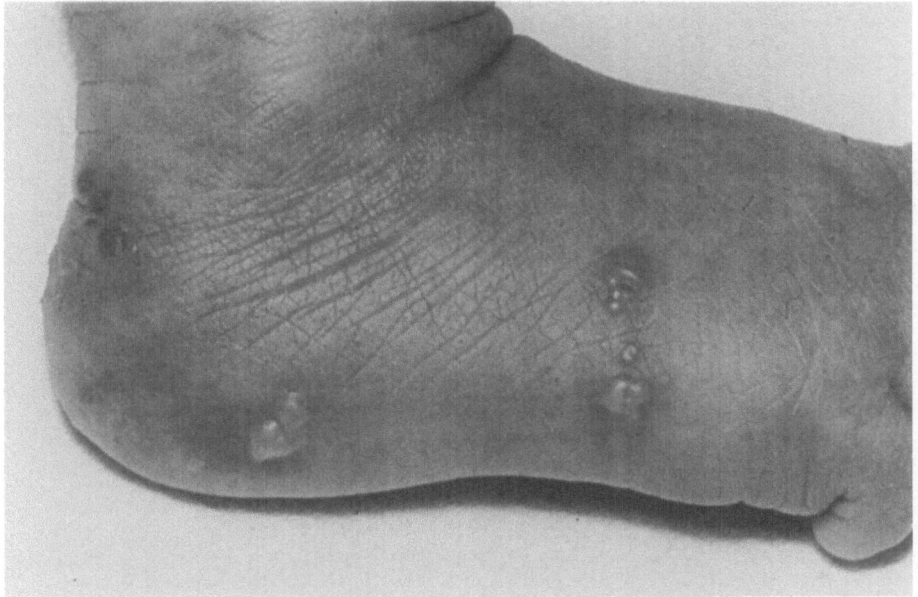

Fig. 5.1. Neonatal herpes: herpetic vesicles on the foot.

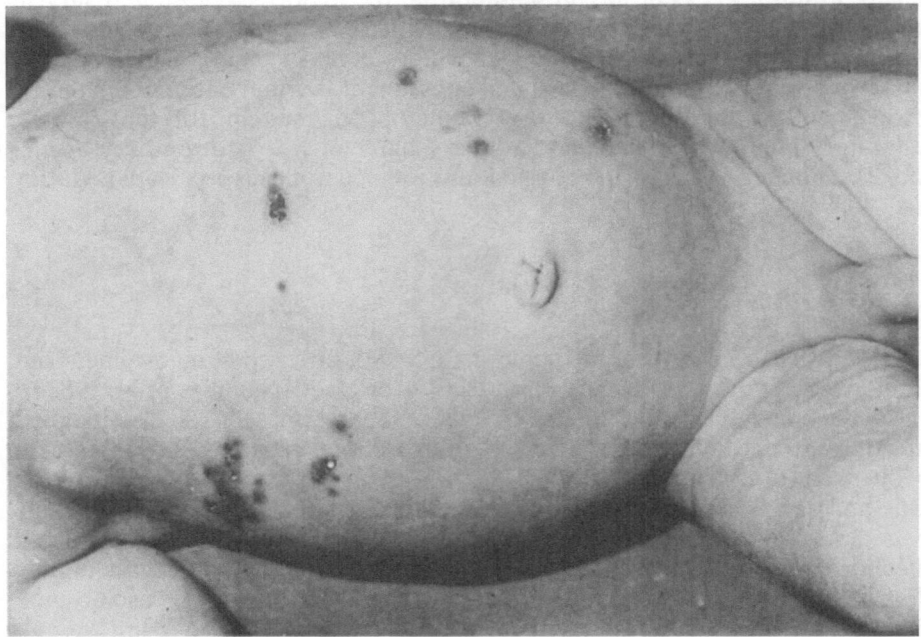

Fig. 5.2. Neonatal herpes: crusted lesions on the abdomen.

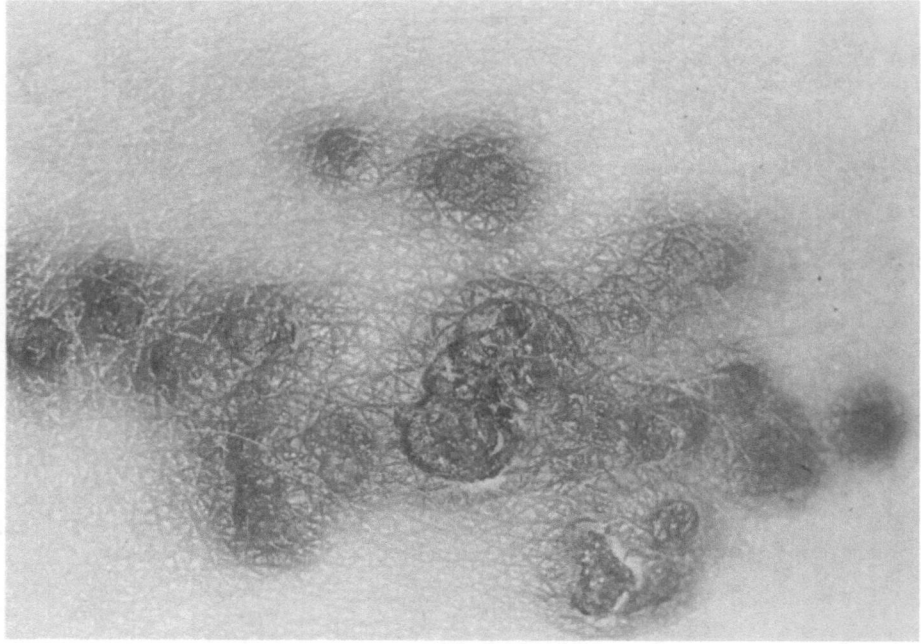

Fig. 5.3. Neonatal herpes: crusted lesions on the abdomen.

erythematous or purphuric maculae, erythema multiforme (Nahmias et al. 1983a), and lesions resembling herpes zoster (Sieber et al, 1966; Music et al. 1971).

Lesions can occur in the oral cavity either alone or in conjunction with disseminated or other forms of localised disease. Ulcerative lesions have been noted on the tongue, buccal mucosa, palate and larynx (Nahmias et al. 1983a).

Ocular herpes, like cutaneous or oral infections, can occur alone or in combination with disseminated or localised disease (Nahmias and Hagler 1972). Virtually any part of the eye may be involved. The commonest presentation is in the form of a blepharoconjunctivitis, with vesicles on the eyelids and surrounding face (Dawson 1984). Other manifestations include choroidoretinitis, conjunctivitis, keratitis, uveitis, retinal dyplasia, microphthalmia and cataracts (Nahmias and Hagler 1972; Nahmias et al. 1983a; Cibis and Burde 1971; Reersted & Hansen 1979). Choroidoretinitis is almost always associated with encephalitis (Hagler et al. 1969).

Mortality and Morbidity

Table 5.3 summarises the mortality and morbidity associated with neonatal herpes. The overall mortality may be as much as 60%. The vast majority of neonates with disseminated infection succumb, as well as a sizeable minority of those with localised CNS disease. The best outcome occurs with localised mouth, skin or eye disease, where the vast majority of individuals survive with no significant long-term sequelae (Nahmias et al. 1983a; Whitley et al. 1980a; Arvin et al. 1982), although some may continue to have localised skin recurrences for many years.

Viral type appears to be important in determining the outcome of neonatal encephalitis (Corey et al. 1988). Neonates infected with HSV 2 have more severe neurological damage, a higher mortality and a greater proportion of survivors with residual neurological problems than those infected with HSV 1.

Table 5.3 Mortality and morbidity associated wth neonatal herpes

Clinical group	% mortality	% survival with sequelae	% survival without sequelae
Disseminated			
No CNS	87–91	2–3	7–10
CNS	71–73	15	12–14
Localised			
CNS	37–41	42–51	12–17
Eye	0	31–39	61–69
Skin	10	21–26	64–69
Mouth	0	0	100
Overall	49–60	19–25	21–26

Based on Nahmias et al. 1983a.

Differential Diagnosis

Certain clinical features of neonatal herpes are reasonably specific. These include skin vesicles or ulcers, oral ulcers and dentritic keratitis. Often, however, the features are less specific. Nahmias et al. (1971) in Atlanta coined the acronym TORCH to cover the group of infectious agents which could infect the neonate. These agents include toxoplasma, rubella, cytomegalovirus and herpes simplex. Other infections causing similar problems include syphilis and a more recent addition to the list, the human immunodeficiency virus (HIV: Shannon and Ammann 1985). All these infections may produce very similar features including CNS problems (encephalitis, microcephaly, hydrocephalitis, intracranial calification and hearing problems), choroidoretinitis, microphthalmia, pneumonia, hepatomegaly, haemolytic anaemia and thrombocytopenia (Nahmias et al. 1971). Pointers towards a diagnosis of neonatal herpes include a history suggestive of HSV in the mother and a more acute onset.

Although the vesicles are relatively specific for HSV infection, particularly when they occur in association with other clinical findings, a number of other conditions that cause vesicles may be confused with herpes. These include varicella, vaccinia, syphilis, staphylococal infection, sepsis due to *Pseudomonas*, *Listeria*, group B streptococci or *Haemophilus influenzae* type B, scabies, candidiasis, toxic epidermal necrolysis, sucking bullae, trauma, neonatal acne, miliaria, acropustulosis of infancy, epidermolysis bullosa and Letterer-Siwe disease (Nahmias et al. 1983a). Other conditions which may need to be excluded include all the infectious causes of encephalitis or septicaemia, hyaline membrane disease and various metabolic defects.

Infection in the Immunosuppressed

Herpes infections can occur in association with a variety of illnesses that cause immunosuppression (Table 5.1). The clinical spectrum ranges from asymptomatic infection to disseminated visceral infection:

Asymptomatic
Localised
   Orolabial
   Genital
   Perianal/anal
Chronic progressive mucocutaneous: orolabial/genital/perianal
Acute mucocutaneous progression: orolabial, genital/perianal
Disseminated visceral infection
   Oesophagus
   Lower respiratory tract infection
   Liver
   Adrenals

HSV is occasionally isolated from oral to genital secretions in asymptomatic individuals whether they are immunosuppressed or not. The only clinical significance of such a finding in the setting of immune depression is to warn the clinician to be on the lookout for subsequent clinically apparent disease.

Infections localised to the lips, genitals or perianal area also occur and, as in immunocompetent individuals, these are usually short lived, self-limiting and

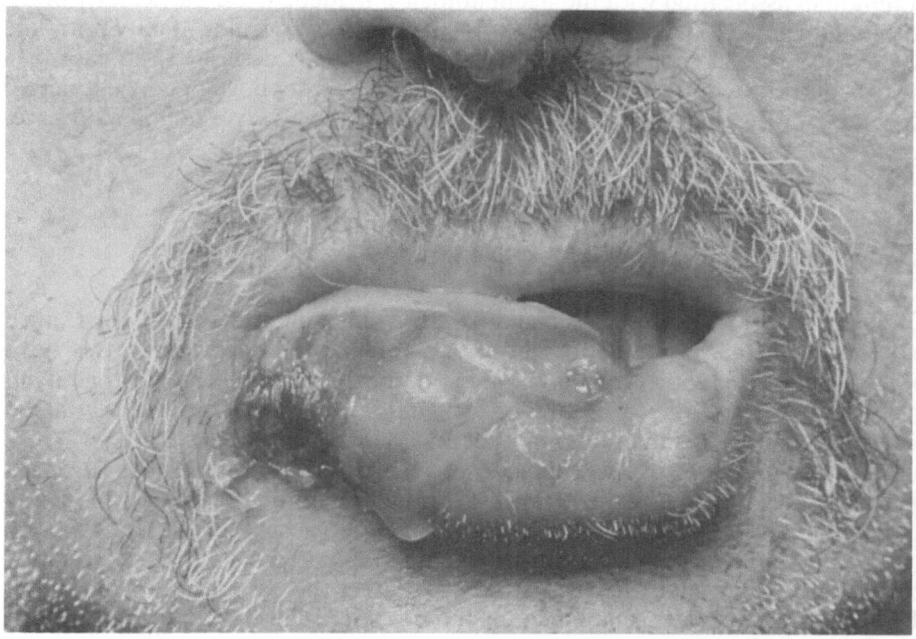

Fig. 5.4. Chronic progressive cutaneous herpes. Severe swelling and ulceration associated with HSV recurrence in a patient with leukaemia.

heal normally. On occasion, however, these relapses may be prolonged and occur with greater frequency.

Chronic Progressive Cutaneous Infections

Localised lesions that fail to heal may become larger and form deeper and necrotic ulcers. Such lesions have been described on the lips (Fig. 5.4), face, genitalia and buttocks and perianal area (Muller et al. 1972; Logan et al. 1971; Siegal et al. 1981; Schneidman et al. 1979). These ulcers appear to be associated with profound immunosuppression, as seen in patients with leukaemias or lymphomas, particularly those on chemotherapy. In patients with the acquired immune deficiency syndrome (AIDS) progressive cutaneous ulceration in the perianal area may be the presenting complaint (Siegal et al. 1981). The spectrum of HSV infection seen with AIDS is described below.

Acute Mucocutaneous Dissemination

Muller et al. (1972) described four cases where HSV infection presented as a widespread disseminated cutaneous problem and in some patients herpes resembled those cases seen in association with various dermatoses (see below). Similar cases have been described by other workers and appear to be particularly common in association with the haematological malignancies, particularly in the terminal phases (Lynfield et al. 1969; Rendtorff and Fowinkle 1965; Smith and Melnick 1962; Solomon 1961). St Geme et al. (1970) described the case of a 3-year-old-boy with Wiskott–Aldrich syndrome, who developed generalised disseminated herpes. The description of the lesions was very similar to cases associated with malignancy.

Visceral Infections

Dissemination to multiple organs may occur if the patient has a viraemia. Such patients are usually immunocompromised (see p. 80); however, cases have been described in otherwise apparently normal individuals (Whorton et al. 1983), and in association with pregnancy where primary HSV has disseminated and resulted in the death of both mother and foetus (Peacock and Sarubbi 1983). Organs that may be involved include the liver, lungs, oesophagus, adrenals, pancreas, the small and large bowel, the kidneys and the bone marrow (Corey and Spear 1986). There have been reports of HSV causing idiopathic thrombo-cytopenia (Whittaker and Hardson 1978) and monoarticular arthritis (Friedman et al. 1980). Occasionally herpes may involve either the oesophagus, the lungs or the liver, without evidence of infection in other visceral organs.

Herpetic Oesophagitis

Herpetic involvement of the oesophagus commonly occurs in association with disseminated visceral disease (Montgomerie et al. 1969; Berg 1955; Taylor et al. 1981; Raga et al. 1984). However, the condition can occur as the sole manifestation of infection in patients with malignancy. Recently several cases have been described in apparently normal individuals (Depew et al. 1977; Owensby and Stammer 1978; Springer et al. 1979; Solammadevi and Patward-han 1982; Deshmukh et al. 1984; DeGaeta et al. 1985). The clinical features include dysphagia and substernal chest pain, and endoscopic examination reveals multiple ulcers or plaques in the mid or distal oesophagus. The ulcers are often very extensive, with a greyish-white exudate and an erythematous halo. Barium swallow shows multiple superficial ulcers or plaques (Levine et al. 1981; Shortsleeve et al. 1981). Clinically, radiologically and endoscopically the condi-tion may be confused with candidal oesophagitis (DeGaeta et al. 1985), cytomegalovirus oesophagitis, thermal injury or radiation injury following ingestion of corrosive substance (Corey and Spear 1986). In patients with normal immunity the ulceration resolves with no residual problems.

Infection of the Lower Respiratory Tract

The entire respiratory epithelium from the nasal and oral mucosa to the alveoli can be infected with HSV (Graham and Snell 1983). The majority of respiratory infections occur in immunocompromised patients; however, patients who have suffered from severe burns may also develop herpetic infections of the lower respiratory tract (Foley et al. 1970; Nash and Foley 1970) and similar problems have been seen following intubation, and associated with the adult respiratory distress syndrome (Tuxen et al. 1983). Studies in bone marrow transplant recipients suggest the HSV causes 6%–8% of the cases of interstitial pneumonia (Ramsey et al. 1982). Many patients will have evidence of visceral involvement (Graham and Snell 1983) and bacterial or fungal superinfection is common (Foley et al. 1970).

Patients with tracheal involvement present with various symptoms including dyspnoea, cough, hoarseness and haemoptysis (Graham and Snell 1983; Foley et al. 1970): bronchoscopy will reveal areas of ulceration or inflammatory membrane formation. Where the disease involves the bronchioles or alveoli, or causes a localised or diffuse pneumonia, symptoms include dyspnoea and cough.

Hepatitis

Post-mortem studies in patients with disseminated HSV infection have shown that involvement of the liver is common (Becker et al. 1968; Raga et al. 1984). The clinical features include fever, hepatomegaly, occasional jaundice and rapid elevation of bilirubin and liver enzymes. The total white cell count is often below 4000 mm^{-3} (Walker et al. 1981; Becker et al. 1968; Raga et al. 1984; Flewett et al. 1969). Without treatment, the condition is rapidly fatal from either liver failure or disseminated intravascular coagulation, or because of involvement of other viscera (Walker et al. 1981; Taylor et al. 1981). Liver biopsy reveals multiple areas of focal necrosis with typical viral intranuclear inclusions in peripheral hepatocytes. Inflammatory response is minimal and is confined to the portal tracts and around the areas of focal necrosis (see Chap. 6) (Flewett et al. 1969; Raga et al. 1984).

Infections in Patients with HIV Infection

In common with other disorders causing profound immune depression, patients with HIV infection may have severe life-threatening herpes infections. However, the full clinical spectrum of conditions due to HSV has been described including mouth ulcers (Quinnan et al. 1984; Barr and Torosian 1986), genital herpes (Clumek et al. 1984), perianal and oral herpes (Siegal et al. 1981; Valle et al. 1985; Mildvan et al. 1982), and HSV encephalitis (Levy et al. 1985). In addition, HSV has been isolated from numerous other organs including the eyes, lungs, oesophagus and bowel (Mildvan et al. 1982; Gold 1985). However, the significance of HSV isolation in the absence of clinical disease is unclear.

Severe persistent perianal herpes is a particular problem amongst homosexual males with AIDS, occurring in up to 13% of cases (Gold 1985). In our experience, the condition often commences as recurrent perianal herpes, which over a period of time becomes more frequent and more persistent. Often, by the time these patients present, the area of ulceration is very extensive, there is a spiking fever, bleeding may be a feature and weight loss is common (Fig. 5.5). Some patients have diarrhoea and an ulcerative proctitis. Other associated opportunistic infections often occur concurrently and some patients may have herpes at other sites, for example around the mouth (Siegal et al. 1981; Mildvan

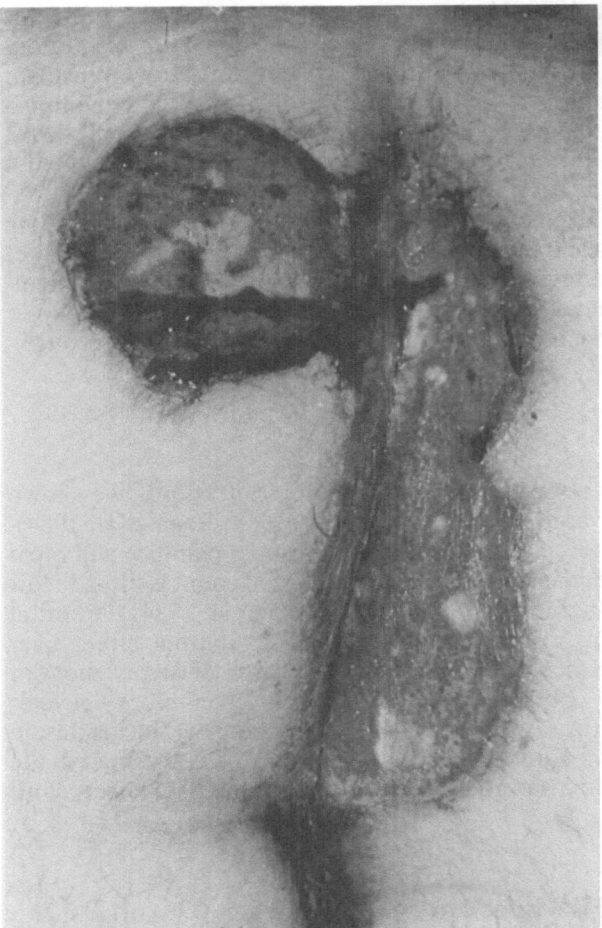

Fig. 5.5. Extensive perianal ulceration due to HSV in a patient with AIDS.

et al 1982). In African patients with AIDS, most of whom are heterosexual, herpes takes the form of persistent mucocutaneous genital herpes (Clumeck et al. 1984). Herpes does not appear to be important in paediatric AIDS patients (Shannon and Ammann 1985), presumably because the majority will not have had previous exposure to HSV.

Herpes encephalitis has been described in patients with AIDS, although it has been suggested that HSV produces a mild diffuse encephalitis in the presence of immunodeficiency and that the more profound the depression the less the inflammation and the more chronic the disease (Levy et al. 1985; Price et al. 1973; Hotson and Pedley 1976; Pitlik et al. 1983). Indeed, in some AIDS patients with profound immunodepression but no obvious neurological illness, HSV has been isolated from the brain post mortem (Levy et al. 1985).

Visceral disseminated HSV infection does not appear to be a major problem in patients with AIDS, although the condition has been reported in terminal patients with multiple infections (Snider et al. 1983).

Infection in Association with Dermatological Conditions

HSV infections are known to complicate several dermatological disorders including atopic eczema (Wheeler et al. 1966), pemphigus (Ogilvie et al. 1983), Darier's disease (Higgins and Crow 1973), pemphigus foliaceous (Silverstein and Burnett, 1967), ichthyosis vulgaris (Verbov et al. 1972) and congenital ichthyosiform erythroderma (Fitzgerald and Booker 1951). Severe HSV infection in association with dermatological complaints has been called eczema herpeticum or Kaposi's varicelliform eruption.

A report by David and Longson (1985) showed that at least 6% of children with atopic eczema develop infection due to HSV. The majority of infections are due to HSV 1 (Leyden and Baker 1979) and usually present as primary infections (Atherton and Marshall 1982; David and Longson 1985). In these patients, the infection is often severe, prolonged and possibly life-threatening. Individuals (usually children) present with high fever, extensive eczema (involving up to 90% of the skin surface) and herpetic vesicles over large areas of the body, including those involved with eczema as well as apparently normal skin (Figs. 5.6, 5.7. and 5.8). The vesicles are fragile and burst to leave large confluent areas of denuded skin (David and Longson 1985). Bacterial infection (usually staphylococcal or streptococcal) is often also present and in these cases the lesions may form pustules. The distinction between herpes and bacterial infection is often difficult, particularly as they often occur together. Visceral dissemination has been described, with death in some cases (Wenner 1944; Mailman et al. 1964). Occasionally death may be due to underlying immune depression as occurs in the Wiskott–Aldrich syndrome (St Geme et al. 1970). Some patients will suffer from recurrences. These are usually of shorter duration, lesser severity and involve smaller areas of skin surface than do the primary attacks (Wheeler et al. 1966; David and Longson 1985).

Kaposi's varicelliform eruption occurs rarely in association with other skin diseases. Verbov et al. (1972) described two adults, with a history of atopic eczema and adult dominant ichthyosis vulgaris, who developed recurrent disseminated herpes infections. The clinical features were similar to those occurring in children with atopic eczema but apparently somewhat milder.

In the other dermatological conditions, pemphigus, Darier's disease, pemphigus foliaceous and congenital ichthyosiform erythroderma, Kaposi's varicelliform eruption takes the form of a severe recrudence of the underlying skin complaint with generalised vesiculation and constitutional symptoms (Ogilvie et al. 1983; Higgins and Crow 1973; Silverstein and Burnett 1967; Fitzgerald and Booker 1951).

HSV infection (both oral and genital) is said to be the commonest precipitating factor for erythema multiforme (EM: Huff et al. 1983; Bean and Quezada 1983; MacDonald and Feiwel 1972; Britz and Sibulkin 1975). The majority of patients with EM have an acute onset of a typical rash (erythematous skin lesions with concentric colour changes) and mucous membrane ulcerations. Most patients will have a single episode; however, recurrences of EM may be associated with recurrent HSV infections (Bean and Quezada 1983). Typically the EM occurs 3 weeks after the recurrent herpes infection (Orton et al. 1984). The pathogenesis of this association remains an enigma but it may be due either

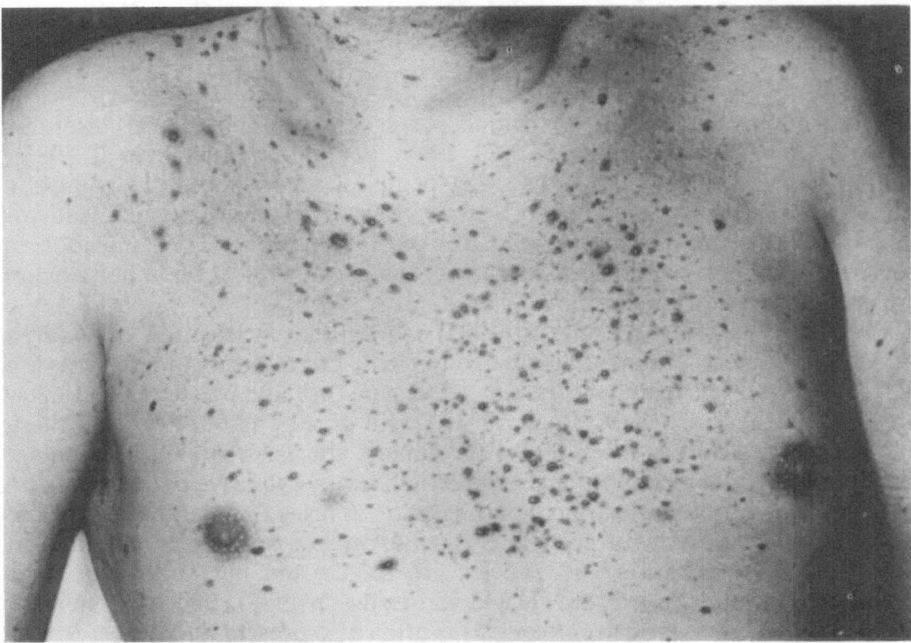

Figs. 5.6, 5.7 and 5.8. Kaposi's varicelliform eruption: disseminated cutaneous herpes associated with atopic eczema.

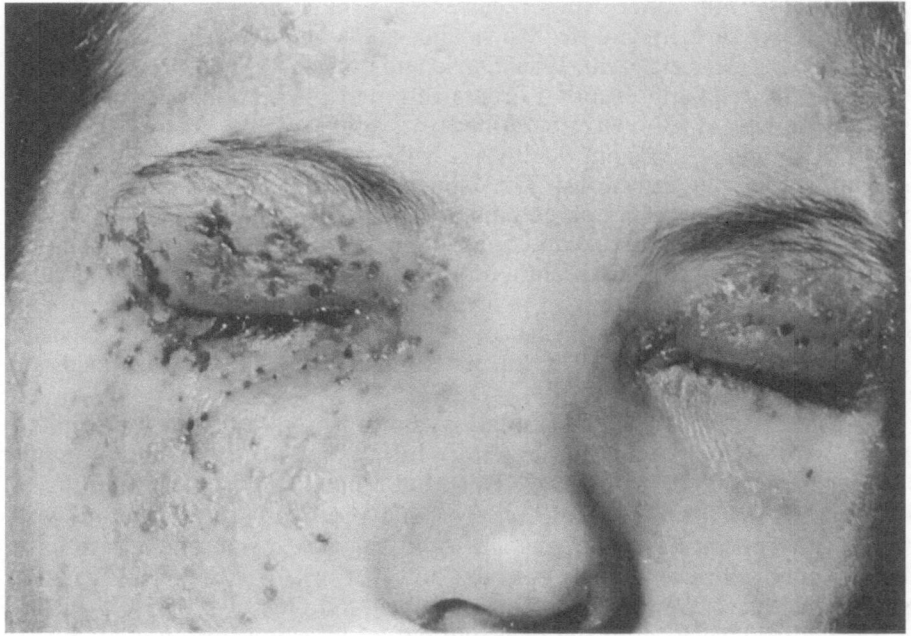

Fig. 5.7.

Fig. 5.8.

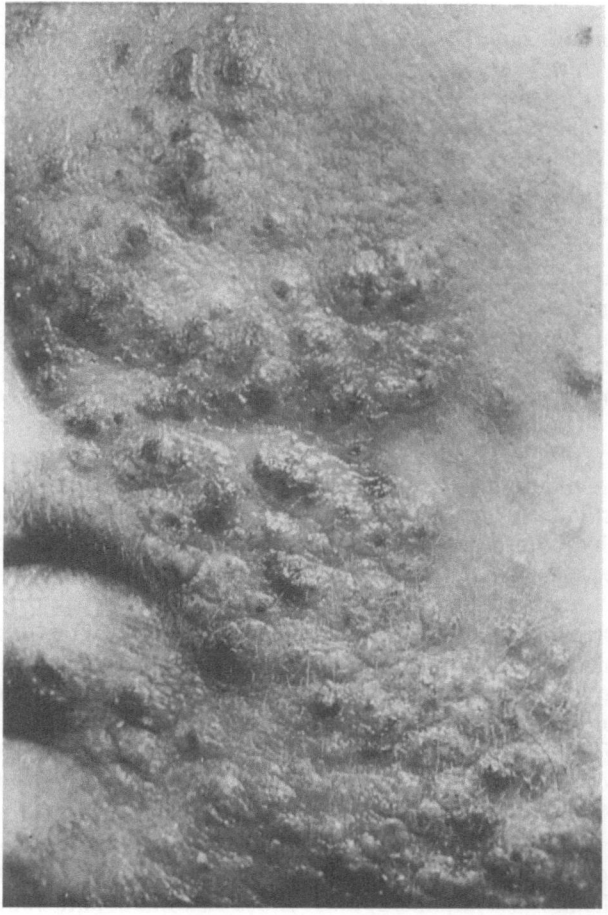

to circulating immune complexes (Kazmierowski and Wuepper 1978; Bushkell et al. 1980) or to deposition of HSV antigen in the skin (Orton et al. 1984).

Encephalitis

Encephalitis is the most feared of all the problems caused by HSV. The reasons for this are that the condition is the commonest cause of fatal encephalitis, that the diagnosis may be difficult and that subsequent treatment may often be unsatisfactory. The disease may affect patients at any age and of both sexes. It is probable that many cases of meningitis and encephalitis are mild, have no long-term sequelae and are often not even clinically suspected let alone investigated (Griffith and Ch'ien 1984).

The onset may be acute or subacute. The majority of patients will have a history of headache, personality changes and altered consciousness or memory loss. Some may have been vomiting or have had grand mal seizure or weakness on one side (Adams and Jennet 1967; Olson et al. 1967; Miller and Ross 1968; Whitley et al. 1982; Skoldenberg et al. 1984; Barza and Pauker 1980). At presentation virtually all patients will be febrile, up to 40% will be comatose or semicomatose and the remainder lethargic. Up to 60% will be disorientated. HSV has a predeliction for the frontal and temporal lobes and focal signs including seizures, hemiparesis, focal numbness or dysphasia occur in virtually all patients (Whitley et al. 1982; Olson et al. 1967). Signs of meningeal irritation are common. Other clinical features occurring in a minority of patients include ataxia, autonomic nervous system dysfunction, cranial nerve palsies and papill-oedema (Whitley et al. 1982). The clinical features in children are often non-specific (McGrossin and Gilbert 1986) and it has been suggested that HSV encephalitis should be suspected in any febrile child with focal seizures or neurological signs and a disturbance in consciousness (Brett 1986).

The differential diagnosis includes brain tumours, abscesses, vascular disease, cryptococcal meningitis, subacute sclerosing panencephalitis, various viral meningitides (including mumps, Epstein–Barr virus, St Louis virus and post-influenzal meningitis), tuberculosis, toxoplasmosis, drug-induced encephalopa-thy, lymphocytic choriomeningitis, Reye's syndrome and acute intermittent porphyria (Lauter 1980; Whitley et al. 1981).

A variety of techniques may be used to confirm the diagnosis; however, all the non-invasive procedures have their limitations. Examination of the CSF is usually unhelpful. Protein level is moderately elevated, the glucose level may be low and the white blood cell count varies from $10~\text{mm}^{-3}$ to $1000~\text{mm}^{-3}$, with a predominance of lymphocytes (Whitley et al. 1982; Griffith and Ch'ien 1984). The CSF white blood cell count is high in the first week, decreasing over the following weeks (Griffith and Ch'ien 1984). Similar changes are seen with other viral and bacterial CNS infections. Although an increase in both serum and CSF HSV antibodies can be documented in most cases, these increases are rarely seen before 10 days of illness and are therefore of limited value when making a diagnosis (Nahmias et al. 1983b; Koskiniemi and Vaheri 1982).

The electroencephalogram (EEG) may be helpful, showing localised periodic lateralising epileptiform discharges or focal slowing over the temporal or frontotemporal regions; however, the EEG may sometimes show only non-specific slowing, indicative of diffuse brain disease (Smith et al. 1975; Upton and Gumpert 1970).

In some patients, increased uptake of isotopes in the temporal lobes may be seen using radionuclide scans; however, in early cases, before swelling of the temporal lobes has occurred, no such changes are apparent (Go et al. 1979; Karlin et al. 1978). Computerised cranial tomography reveals unilateral low density lesions in the region of the temporal lobes in 50%–75% of cases (Dublin and Merten 1977; Enzmann et al. 1978; Ketonen and Koskiniemi 1980). Early reports on the use of magnetic resonance imaging (MRI; Schroth et al. 1987) and single photon emission computed tomography (SPECT; Launes et al. 1988) suggest that both these techniques may be useful in early diagnosis of HSV encephalitis.

Brain biopsy is the most specific method of making a diagnosis of HSV encephalitis and has the advantages of a low complication rate and the possible diagnosis of other potentially treatable conditions (Whitley et al. 1981). Unfor-tunately brain biopsy may be negative in up to half the cases, because an uninfected site was biopsied, or the specimen was not processed and studied correctly, or, as mentioned above, the patient does not have HSV encephalitis (Whitley et al. 1981; Nahmias et al. 1983b). Until the introduction of acyclovir there was a very aggressive lobby advocating the use of brain biopsy in all cases (Whitley et al. 1982; Nahmias et al. 1983b); however, many authors now believe that routine brain biopsy is unnecessary and recommend that acyclovir should be started immediately whilst less invasive investigations are initiated (Anonymous 1986; Brett 1986). When a brain biopsy is taken, histology may reveal perivascular lymphocytic infiltration and cytology may show intranuclear inclusions (see Chap. 6). HSV can be isolated from neuronal tissue or detected using an immunofluorescent stain and monoclonal antibodies (Flewett 1973; Tomlinson et al. 1974; see also Chap. 7).

The prognosis of herpes simplex encephalitis is dismal and without treatment the overall mortality rate is 70%–80% after 30 days, rising to 90% by 6 months (Whitley et al. 1977). The majority of survivors will have a moderate or severe residual neurological impairment (see Chap. 8). The outlook irrespective of therapy is worse in elderly patients and those with impaired levels of consciousness.

Possible Role of HSV in Other Neurological Disorders, Atherosclerosis and Duodenal Ulcers

Other Neurological Disorders

It has been suggested that HSV may be involved in the pathogenesis of various psychiatric and neurological disorders, including temporal lobal epilepsy and multiple sclerosis. The evidence cited includes the observation that HSV is neurotrophic, that some of these complaints are recurrent (Kirchner 1982) and that HSV DNA has been detected in the brain of a small number of patients with chronic psychiatric disorders or temporal lobe epilepsy (Sequiera et al. 1979; Gannicliffe et al. 1985).

Infection with HSV has been shown to produce demyelinisation of the CNS in experimentally infected animals, and this observation has been used to suggest that the virus may be implicated in the causation of multiple sclerosis. HSV has been isolated from the brain of one patient with multiple sclerosis (Gudnadottir et al. 1964) and the CSF of another (Vahlne et al. 1985), but as yet there are no studies looking for evidence of HSV DNA from the demyelinated areas of brains of patients with multiple sclerosis.

The evidence to date is interesting but far from convincing and considerably more information will be required before the role of HSV (if any) in these conditions can be determined.

Atherosclerosis

Chickens with Marek's disease (a conditon caused by a herpes group virus) develop lesions in their arteries that resemble human atherosclerosis, especially when given a high-cholesterol diet (Sprecher and Cappel 1980). This observation has been used to suggest a possible link between HSV and atherosclerosis in humans. Recent studies on human and bovine smooth muscle cells have shown that HSV-infected cells accumulate greater amounts of cholesterol esters and triglycerides than those that are uninfected (Hajjar et al. 1987), suggesting that HSV may be important on the accumulation of lipids and thus in the production of atherosclerosis. However, HSV has not been isolated from atherosclerotic plaques, and patients with atherosclerosis are no more likely to have serological evidence of HSV than anybody else.

Duodenal Ulcer

The evidence possibly linking HSV and duodenal ulcers is a little more substantial. Firstly HSV has been isolated from the vagal ganglia (Warren et al. 1978; Lonsdale et al. 1980), suggesting that HSV may reactivate and recur within the nerves of the digestive tract. Psychological factors have long been considered as important on the pathogenesis of duodenal ulcers, Vagal stimulation (with possible viral reactivation) has been postulated to occur at this time. It has also been shown that patients with duodenal ulcers are more likely to have antibodies to HSV 1 (but not HSV 2) than are control groups (Vestergaard and Rune 1980).

Bell's Palsy

In most cases of lower motor neurone facial palsy (Bell's palsy) no obvious cause or precipating factor can be found, but several recent reports have suggested that there could be a link with HSV (Adour et al. 1978; McCormick 1972; Vahlne et al. 1981; Grout 1977; Wilson 1978; Smith et al. 1987). What is the nature of this link? In some cases it seems to occur with, or soon after, classical labial herpes (Smith et al. 1987; Vahlne et al. 1981), suggesting some direct involvement of the facial nerve in the region of the trigeminal ganglion. Other reports have suggested that HSV may cause demyelination (see above for discussion on multiple sclerosis) at the level of the brain stem, affecting the facial nucleus or facial nerve tracts (Vahlne et al. 1985). The possible mechanisms causing such demyelination are unknown, although the possibility of an auto-immune response has been considered (Smith et al. 1987).

Oral and genital herpes are both very common (see Chap. 4) but Bell's palsy is not, suggesting that the association (if any) is not a very strong one.

References

Adams JH, Jennet WB (1967) Acute necrotising encephalitis: a problem in diagnosis. J Neurol Neurosurg Psychiatry 30: 248–260

Adour KK, Bye FM, Hilsinger RL, Kahn ZM, Sheldon MJ (1978) The true nature of Bell's palsy: analysis of 1000 consecutive patients. Laryngoscope 88: 787–801

Alford CA (1984) Chronic intrauterine and perinatal infections. In: Galasso GJ, Merigan TC, Buchanan RA (eds) Antiviral agents and viral disease of man, 2nd edn. Raven Press, New York, pp 433–486

Anonymous (1986) Herpes simplex encephalitis. Lancet i: 535–536

Arvin AM, Yaeger AS, Bruhn FW, Grossman M (1982) Neonatal herpes simplex infection in the absence of mucocutaneous lesions. J Pediatr 100: 715–721

Atherton DJ, Marshall WC (1982) Eczema herpeticum. Practitioner 226: 971–973

Barr CE, Torosian JP (1986) Oral manifestation in patients with AIDS or AIDS-related complex. Lancet ii: 288

Barza M, Pauker SG (1980) The decision to biopsy, treat, or wait in suspected herpes encephalitis. Ann Intern Med 92: 641–649

Bean SF, Quezada RK (1983) Recurrent oral erythema multiforme: clinical experience with 11 patients. JAMA 249: 2810–2812

Becker WB, Kipps A, McKenzie D (1968) Disseminated herpes simplex virus infection. Am J Dis Child 115: 1–8

Berg JW (1955) Oesophageal herpes: a complication of cancer therapy. Cancer 8: 731–740

Brett EM (1986) Herpes simplex virus encephalitis in children. Br Med J 293: 1388–1389

Britz M, Sibulkin D (1975) Recurrent erythema multiforme and herpes genitalia (type 2). JAMA 233: 812–813

Bushkell LL, Mackel SE, Jordon RE (1980) Erythema multiforme: direct immunofluorescence studies and detection of circulating immune complexes. J Invest Dermatol 74: 372–374

Cibis A, Burde RM (1971) Herpes simplex virus induced congenital cataracts. Arch Ophthalmol 85: 220–223

Clumeck N, Sonnet J, Taelman H (1984) Acquired immunodeficiency syndrome in African patients. N Engl J Med 310: 492–497

Corey L, Spear PG (1986) Infections with herpes simplex viruses. (Second of two parts.) N Engl J Med 314: 749–757

Corey L, Whitley RJ, Stone EF, Mohan K (1988) Difference between herpes simplex virus type 1 and type 2 neonatal encephalitis in neurological outcome. Lancet i: 1–4

David TJ, Longson M (1985) Herpes simplex infections in atopic eczema. Arch Dis Child 60: 338–343

Dawson CR (1984) Ocular herpes simplex virus infections. Clin Dermatol 2: 56–66

DeGaeta L, Levine MS, Guglielmi GE, Raffensperger EC, Laufer I (1985) Herpes esophagitis in an otherwise healthy patient. AJR 144: 1205–1206

Depew WT, Prentice RG, Beck IT, Blakeman JM, DaCosta LR (1977) Herpes simplex ulcerative esophagitis in a healthy subject. Am J Gastroenterol 68: 381–385

Deshmukh M, Shah R, MacCallum RW (1984) Experience with herpes esophagitis in otherwise healthy patients. Am J Gastroenterol 79: 173–176

Dublin AB, Merten DF (1977) Computerised tomography in the evaluation of herpes simplex encephalitis. Radiology 125: 133–134

Enzmann DR, Ranson B, Norman D et al. (1978) Computed tomography of herpes simplex encephalitis. Radiology 129: 419–425

Fitzgerald WC, Booker AP (1951) Congenital ichthyosiform erythroderma. A case report of cases in siblings, one complicated by Kaposi's varicelliform eruption. Arch Derm Syph 64: 611–619

Flewett, TH (1973) The rapid diagnosis of herpes encephalitis. Postgrad Med J 49: 398–400

Flewett TH, Parker RGF, Philip WM (1969) Acute hepatitis due to herpes simplex virtus in the adult. J Clin Pathol 22: 60–66

Florman AL, Gershon AA, Blackett PR, Nahmias AJ (1973) Intrauterine infection with herpes simplex virus. Resultant congenital malformations. JAMA 225: 129–132

Foley FD, Greenwald KA, Nash G, Pruitt BA (1970) Herpesvirus infection in burned patients. N Engl J Med 282: 652–656

Friedman HM, Pincus T, Gibilisco P, et al. (1980) Acute monoarticular arthritis caused by herpes simplex virus and cytomegalovirus. Am J Med 69: 241–247

Gannicliffe A, Saldanha JA, Itzhaki RF, Sutton RNP (1985) Herpes simplex viral DNA in temporal lobe epilepsy. Lancet i: 214–215

Go RT, Yousef MMA, Jacoby C G (1979) The rate of radionuclide brain imaging and computerised tomography in the early diagnosis of herpes. J Comput Tomogr 3: 286–296

Gold JWM (1985) Clinical spectrum of infection in patients with HTLV–III associated disease. Cancer Res 45: 4652–4654

Graham BS, Snell JD (1983) Herpes simplex virus infection of the adult lower respiratory tract. Medicine (Baltimore) 62: 384–393

Griffith JF, Ch'ien LT (1984) Viral infection of the central nervous system. In: Galasso GJ, Merigan TC, Buchanan RA (eds) Antiviral agents and viral diseases of man, 2nd edn. Raven Press, New York, pp 399–432

Grout P (1977) Bell's palsy and herpes simplex. Br Med J 2: 829–830

Gudnadottir M, Helgadottir H, Bjarnason O, Jonsdottir K (1964) Virus isolated from the brain of a patient with multiple sclerosis. Exp Neurol 9: 85–95

Hagler WS, Walters DV, Nahmias AJ (1969) Ocular involvement in neonatal herpes simplex virus infection. Arch Opthalmol 82: 169–176

Hajjar DP, Pomerantz KB, Falcone DJ, Weksler BB, Grant AJ (1987) Herpes simplex virus infection of human arterial cells. Implications in arteriosclerosis. J Clin Invest 80: 1317–1321

Higgins PG, Crow KD (1973) Recurrent Kaposi's varicelliform eruption in Darier's disease. Br J Dermatol 88: 391–394

Honig PJ, Brown D (1982) Congenital herpes simplex virus infection initially resembling epidermolysis bullosa. J Pediatr 101: 958–959

Hotson JR, Pedley TA (1976) The neurological complications of cardiac transplantation. Brain 99: 673–694

Huff JC, Weston WL, Tonnesen MG (1983) Erythema multiforme: a critical review of characteristics, diagnostic criteria, and causes. J Am Acad Dermatol 8: 763–775

Jenista JA (1984) Perinatal herpesvirus infections. In: Amstey MS (ed) Virus infection in pregnancy. Grune and Stratton Inc., Orlando, F L, pp 69–79

Karlin CA, Robinson RG, Hinthorn DR, et al. (1978) Radionuclide imaging in herpes simplex encephalitis. Radiology 126: 181–184

Kazmierowski JA, Wuepper KD (1978) Erythema multiforme: immune complex vasculitis of the superficial cutaneous microvasculture. J Invest Dermatol 71: 366–369

Ketonen K, Koskiniemi M (1980) Computed tomography appearance of herpes simplex encephalitis. Clin Radiol 31: 161–165

Kirchner H (1982) Immunobiology of infection with herpes simplex virus. Karger, Basel.

Koskiniemi ML, Vaheri A (1982) Diagnostic value of cerebrospinal fluid antibodies in herpes simplex virus encephalitis. J Neurol Neurosurg Psychiatry 45: 239–242

Launes J, Nikkinen P, Lindroth L, Brownell A–L, Liewendahl K, Iivanainen M (1988) Diagnosis of acute herpes simplex encephalitis by brain perfusion single photon emission computed tomography. Lancet i: 1188–1191

Lauter CB (1980) Herpes simplex encephalitis. A great clinical challenge. Ann Intern Med 93: 696–697

Levine MS, Laufer I, Kressel HY, Friedman HM (1981) Herpes esophagitis. A J R 136: 836–866

Levy RM, Bredesen DE, Rosenblum ML (1985) Neurological manifestation of the acquired immunodeficiency syndrome (AIDS). Experience of UCSF and review of the literature. J Neurosurg 62: 475–495

Leyden JJ, Baker DA (1979) Localised herpes simplex infections in atopic dermatitis. Arch Dermatol 115: 311–312

Logan WS, Tindall JP, Elson ML (1971) Chronic cutaneous herpes simplex. Arch Dermatol 103: 606–614

Lonsdale DM, Brown SM, Lang J, Subak-Sharpe JH, Koprowski H, Warnen KG (1980) Variations in herpes simplex virus isolated from human ganglia and a study of clonal variation in HSV 1. Ann N Y Acad Sci 354: 291–308

Lynfield YL, Farhangi M, Runnels JL (1969) Generalised herpes simplex complicating lymphoma. JAMA 207: 944–945

MacDonald A, Feiwel M (1972) Isolation of herpes virus from erythema multiforme. Br Med J 2: 570–571

Mailman CJ, Miranda JL, Speck A (1964) Recurrent eczema herpeticum. Arch Dermatol 89: 815–818

McCormick DP (1972) Herpes simplex virus as a cause of Bell's palsy. Lancet i: 937–939

McGrossin DB, Gilbert GL (1986) Herpes simplex virus encephalitis in children. Med J Aus 144: 711–713

Mildvan D, Mathur U, Enslow RW, et al. (1982) Opportunistic infection and immune deficiency in homosexual men. Ann Intern Med 96: 700–704

Miller JD, Ross CA (1968) Encephalitis: a 4 year survey. Lancet i: 1121–1126

Monif GRG, Kellner KR, Donnelly WH (1985) Congenital herpes simplex type II infection. Am J Obstet Gynecol 152: 1000–1002

Montgomerie JZ, Becroft DMO, Croxson MC, Doak PB, North JDK (1969) Herpes simplex virus infection after renal transplantation. Lancet ii: 867–871

Muller SA, Herrman EC, Winkelmann RK (1972) Herpes simplex infection in hematological malignancies. Am J Med 52: 102–114

Music SI, Fine EM, Togo Y (1971) Zoster like disease in the newborn due to herpes simplex virus. N Engl J Med 284: 24–26

Nahmias AJ, Hagler WS (1972) Ocular manifestation of herpes simplex in the newborn (neonatal ocular herpes). Int Ophthalmol Clin 12: 191–213

Nahmias AJ, Alford CA, Korones SB (1970) Infection of the newborn with herpes virus hominis. Adv Paediatr 17: 185–226

Nahmias AJ, Watts K, Stewart J, Flynn W, Hermann K (1971) The TORCH complex: perinatal infection associated with toxoplasma and rubella cytomegalo – and herpes simplex viruses. Pediatr Res 5: 405–406

Nahmias AJ, Keyserling HH, Kerrick G (1983a) Herpes simplex. In: Remington JS, Klein JO (eds) Infectious diseases of the fetus and newborn infant. WB Saunders, Philadelphia, pp 156–190

Nahmias AJ, Whitley RJ, Visintine AN, Takei Y, Alford CAJ (1983b) Collaborative antiviral study group. Herpes simplex virus encephalitis: laboratory evaluations and their diagnostic significance. J Infect Dis 145: 829–836

Nash G, Foley FD (1970) Herpetic infection of the middle and lower respiratory tract. Am J Clin Path 54: 857–863

Ogilvie MM, Kesseler M, Leppard BJ, Goodwin P, White JE (1983) Herpes simplex infections in pemphigus: an indication for urgent viral studies and specific antiviral therapy. Br J Dermatol 109: 611–613

Olson LC, Buescher EL, Artenstein MS, Parkman PD (1967) Herpesvirus infection of the human central nervous system. N Engl J Med 227: 1271–1277

Orton PW, Huff JC, Toneson MG, Weston WC (1984) Detection of a herpes viral antigen in skin lesions of erythema multiforme. Ann Intern Med 101: 48–50

Owensby LC, Stammer JL (1978) Esophagitis associated with herpes simplex infection in an immunocompetent host. Gastroenterology 74: 1305–1306

Peacock JE Jr, Sarubbi FA (1983) Disseminated herpes simplex virus infection during pregnancy. Obstet Gynecol Suppl 61: 13s–18s

Pitlik SD, Fainstein V, Bolivar R, et al. (1983) Spectrum of central nervous system complications in homosexual men with acquired immune deficiency syndrome. J Infect Dis 148: 771–772

Price R, Chernik NL, Horta-Barbosa L, et al. (1973) Herpes simplex encephalitis in an anergic patient. Am J Med: 54: 222–228

Quinnan GV, Masur H, Rook AH, et al. (1984) Herpesvirus infection in the acquired immune deficiency syndrome. JAMA 252: 72–77

Raga J, Chrystal V, Coovadia HM (1984) Usefulness of clinical features and liver biopsy in diagnosis of disseminated herpes simplex infection. Arch Dis Child 59: 820–824

Ramsey PG, Fife KH, Hackman RC, Meyers JP, Corey L (1982) Herpes simplex virus pneumonia: clinical virologic and pathologic features in 20 patients. Ann Intern Med 97: 813–820

Reersted P, Hansen B (1979) Chorioretinitis of the newborn with herpes simplex virus type 1: report of a case. Acta Opthalmol 57: 1096–1100

Rendtorff RC, Fowinkle EW (1965) Herpes simplex skin lesions simulating smallpox. JAMA 192: 998–1000

Schroth G, Gawehn J, Thron A, Vallbracht A, Voigt K (1987) Early diagnosis of herpes simplex encephalitis by MRI. Neurology 37: 179–183

Sequiera LW, Carrasco LH, Carry A, Jennings LC, Lord MA, Sutton RNP (1979) Detection of herpes simplex viral genome in brain tissue. Lancet ii: 609–612

Shannon KM, Ammann AJ (1985) Acquired immune deficiency syndrome in childhood. J Pediatr 106: 332–342

Schneidman DW, Barr RJ, Graham JH (1979) Chronic cutaneous herpes simplex. JAMA 241: 592–594

Shortsleeve MJ, Gauvin GP, Gardner RC, Greenberg MS (1981) Herpetic esophagitis. Radiology 141: 611–617

Sieber OF Jr, Fulginiti VA, Brazie J, Umlauf HJ Jr (1966) In utero infection of the fetus by herpes simplex virus. J Pediatr 69: 30–34

Siegal FP, Lopez C, Hammer GS, et al. (1981) Severe acquired immunodeficiency in male homosexuals, manifested by chronic perianal ulcerative herpes simplex lesions. N Engl J Med 305: 1439–1444

Silverstein EH, Burnett JW (1967) Kaposi's varicelliform eruption complicating pemphigus folia-
    ceous. Arch Dermatol 95: 214–216
Sköldenberg B, Forsgren M, Alestig K, et al. (1984) Acyclovir versus vidarabine in herpes simplex
    encephalitis. Randomised multicentre study in consecutive Swedish patients. Lancet ii: 707–711
Smith JB, Westmoreland BF, Reagan TJ, Sandok BA (1975) A distinctive clinical EEG profile on
    herpes simplex encephalitis. Mayo Clin Proc 50: 469–474
Smith KO, Melnick JL (1962) Recognition and quantitation of herpes virus particles in human
    vesicular lesions. Science 137: 543–544
Smith MD, Scott GM, Rom S and Patou G (1987) Herpes simplex virus and facial palsy. J Infect 15:
    259–261
Snider WO, Simpson DM, Nielsen S, Gold JWM, Metroka CE, Posner JB (1983) Neurological
    complications of acquired immune deficiency syndrome: analysis of 50 patients. Ann Neurol 14:
    403–418
Solammadevi SV, Patwardhan R (1982) Herpes esophagitis. Am J Gastroenterol 77: 48–50
Solomon M (1961) Herpes simplex virus from skin lesions of myelogenous leukaemia. Arch Intern
    Med 107: 100–104
South MA, Tompkins WAF, Morris CR, Rawls WE (1969) Congenital malformation of the central
    nervous system associated with genital (type 2) herpes virus. J Pediatr 75: 13–18
Sprecher S, Cappel R (1980) Association of herpesviruses with arteriosclerosis and neuropsychiatric
    disorders. In: Nahmias AJ, Dowdle WR, Schinazi R (eds) An interdisciplinary perspective.
    Elsevier, New York, pp 45–47
Springer DL, DaCosta LR, Beck IT (1979) A syndrome of acute self limiting ulcerative esophagitis
    in young adults probably due to herpes simplex virus. Dig Dis Sci 24: 535–539
St Geme JW, Prince JT, Burke BA, et al. (1970) Impaired cellular resistance to herpes simplex virus
    in Wiskott–Aldrich syndrome. N Engl J Med 273: 229–234
Stagno S, Whitley RJ (1985) Herpesvirus infection in pregnancy. Part II. Herpes simplex virus and
    varicella zoster infections. N Engl J Med 313: 1327–1330
Sullivan–Bolyai J, Hull HF, Wilson C, Corey L (1983) Neonatal herpes simplex virus infection in
    King County, Washington. Increasing incidence and epidemiologic correlates. JAMA 250:
    3059–3062
Taylor RJ, Saul SH, Dowling JN, Hakala TR, Peel RL, Ho M (1981) Primary disseminated herpes
    simplex infection with fulminant hepatitis following renal transplantation. Arch Intern Med 141:
    1519–1521
Tomlinson AH, Chinn IJ, MacCallum FO (1974) Immunofluorescence staining for the diagnosis of
    herpes encephalitis. J Clin Pathol 27: 495–499
Tuxen DV, Cude JF, McDonald MI, Buchanan MRC, Clark RJ, Pain MCF (1983) Herpes simplex
    virus from the lower respiratory tract in adult respiratory distress syndrome. Am Rev Respir Dis
    126: 416–419
Upton A, Gumpert J (1970) Electroencephalography in diagnosis of herpes simplex encephalitis.
    Lancet i: 650–652
Vahlne A, Edström S, Arstila P, et al. (1981) Bell's palsy and herpes simplex virus. Arch
    Otolaryngol 107: 79–81
Vahlne A, Edström S, Hanner P, Anderson O, Svennerholm B, Lycke E (1985) Possible association
    of herpes simplex virus infection with demyelinating disease. Scand J Infect Dis 47 [suppl]: 16–21
Valle S, Saxinger C, Ranki A, et al. (1985) Diversity of clinical spectrum of HTLV–III infection.
    Lancet i: 301–304
Verbov J, Munro DP, Miller A (1972) Recurrent eczema herpeticum associated with ichthyosis
    vulgaris. Br J Derm 86: 638–640
Vestergaard BF, Rune SJ (1980) Type-specific herpes-simplex-virus antibodies in patients with
    recurrent duodenal ulcer. Lancet i: 1273–1275
Walker DP, Longson M, Lawler W, Mallick NP, Davies JS, Johnson RWG (1981) Disseminated
    herpes simplex virus infection with hepatitis in an adult renal transplant recipient. J Clin Pathol
    34: 1044–1046
Warren KG, Brown SM, Wroblewska Z, Gilden D, Koprowski H, Subak-Sharpe J (1978) Isolation
    of latent herpes simplex virus from the superior cervical and vagus ganglions of human beings.
    N Negl J Med 298: 1068–1070
Warren KG, Koprowski H, Lonsdale DM, Brown SM, Subak-Sharpe JH (1979) The polypeptide
    and DNA restriction enzyme profiles of spontaneous isolates of herpes simplex virus type 1 from
    explants of human trigeminal superior cervical and vagus ganglia. J Gen Virol 43: 151–171
Wenner HA (1944) Complications of infantile eczema caused by the virus of herpes simplex. Am J
    Dis Child 4: 247–264

Wheeler CE, Abele DC, Hill C (1966) Eczema herpeticum primary and recurrent. Arch Dermatol 93: 162–173

Whitley RJ, Soong S-J, Dolin R et al. (1977) Adenine arabinoside therapy of biopsy-proved herpes simplex virus encephalitis. National Institute of Allergy and Infectious Diseases collaborative antiviral study. N Engl J Med 297: 289–294

Whitley RJ, Nahmias AJ, Soong S-J, Galasso GJ, Fleming CL, Alford CA (1980a) Vidarabine therapy of neonatal herpes simplex virus infection. Pediatrics 66: 495–501

Whitley RJ, Nahmias AJ, Visintine AM, Fleming CL, Alford CA (1980b) The natural history of herpes simplex virus of mother and newborn. Pediatrics 66: 489–494

Whitley RJ, Soong S-J, Hirsch MS, et al. (1981) Herpes simplex encephalitis vidarabine therapy and diagnostic problems. N Engl J Med 304: 313–318

Whitley RJ, Soong S-J, Linneman C, Liu C, Pazin G, Alford CA (1982) Herpes simplex encephalitis. JAMA 247: 317–320

Whittaker JA, Hardson JE (1978) Severe thrombocytopenia after generalised herpes simplex virus 2 (HSV-2) infection. South Med J 71: 864–865

Whorton CM, Thomas DM, Denham SW (1983) Fatal systemic herpes simplex virus type 2 infection in a healthy young woman. South Med J 76: 81–83

Wilson JB (1978) Bell's palsy and herpes simplex. Br Med J 2: 704

Chapter 6

Pathology and Pathogenesis

Pathology

Introduction

There are two separate and distinct outcomes following cellular infection with herpes simplex: (1) a productive infection (see Chap. 1) with active viral replication, occurring first in epithelial cells and resulting in ultimate cell death; and (2) a non-productive (or latent) infection, occurring in nerve cells (see Chap. 2). The productive infection causes most of the clinical symptoms and signs associated with herpes, from the most trivial cutaneous lesions to widespread disseminated illness seen in immunocompromised patients (see Chaps. 4 and 5). The latent (non-productive) infection does not itself cause any pathological changes but is responsible for the reactivation characteristic of HSV infections.

Pathological Changes Associated with Productive Infection

The basic pathological changes that occur during productive infection in the epithelium are the same whether the lesions are occurring on the lips, mouth, genital area, perianal area or indeed any other area of epidermis or mucosa. The pathological process involved with both primary and recurrent infection is identical. Macroscopically the first change is erythema followed within a few hours by fluid-filled vesicles or blisters; these rupture within a few days to leave shallow ulcers with a necrotic base. On moist surfaces the ulcers heal from the edge without crusting, whereas on dry skin surfaces the ulcers form scabs or crusts and then heal (see Chap. 4).

Histopathology (Fig. 6.1)

When only erythema is present (i.e. the earliest lesions) the epidermis is intact and there may be proliferate changes in the epidermis. The infiltrate consists

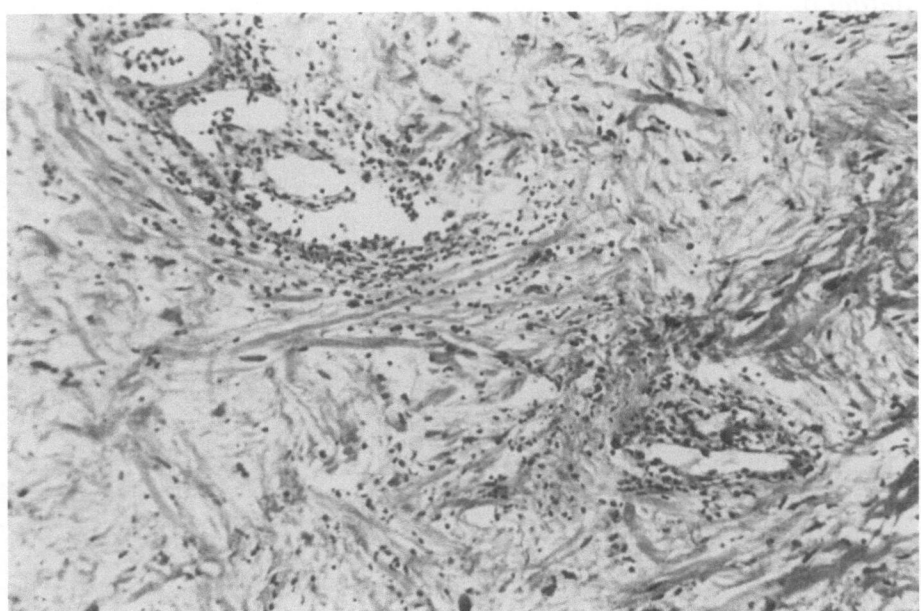

Fig. 6.1. Histopathology of subcutaneous HSV infection. Marked round-cell infiltrate with areas of superficial necrosis. (Courtesy of Dr D Katz.) (× 90).

mainly of lymphocytes and neutrophils (Haber et al. 1980). As the lesions progress, the cells begin to degenerate and vesicles appear within the epidermis. The infected cells lose their intracellular prickles (acantholysis), and swell. The cytoplasm becomes eosinophilic and the cell nuclei become multiple (see cytology below). Eosinophilic nuclear inclusions, usually single and surrounded by a halo, can be seen (Cowdry 1934). Similar inclusions may be seen with several other viral infections including varicella zoster, cytomegalovirus and in subacute sclerosing panencephalitis. Ultimately, the surface epithelium ulcerates. In these advanced lesions, cell debri, macrophages and occasional lymphocytes are present (Cunningham et al. 1985). Lesions heal by regrowth of the epithelium. A mononuclear infiltrate may be present in the underlying dermis.

Recent immunohistological studies have shown that most of the cells constituting the infiltrate are T lymphocytes and macrophages. In early lesions, T helper cells are common, whilst in later lesions monocytes and macrophages predominate (Cunningham et al. 1985).

The histopathological changes associated with HSV skin or mucous membrane infection cannot be differentiated from those produced by varicella zoster.

The cytological changes associated with HSV can be used for diagnosis (see Chap. 7). Suitable material to examine includes scrapings from denuded vesicles and from the margins of ulcers or crusts (Naib 1984). Such material can be taken from any anatomical site, including exfoliated cells from the genital tract, or perioral region, bronchial washings, oesophageal scrapings or transitional cells in urine specimens. After fixation, slides can be stained with a variety of stains including Giemsa, Wright's or Papanicolaou's. The infected cells go through a series of changes (Naib 1966). Newly infected cells have a small amount of cytoplasm and an enlarged nucleus, the chromatin may be pushed to the periphery by the replicating virus, The nuclear membrane is thickened and the nucleus disintegrates. Sometimes, before disappearing, the nuclei may enlarge. Naib (1984) has commented that these early changes may be mistaken for cancer. As the infection progresses there is a syncytial merging of infected cells, with the production of mulinucleated cells, first with bland nuclei, but later on with well-demarcated, granular, single eosinophilic inclusions (Fig. 6.2). These inclusions are pathognomonic for herpes simplex.

Pathology of Different Anatomical Sites

Cervix

The typical histological changes described above can be seen on cervical biopsy and are found at the edge of ulcers most often at or near the squamocolumnar junction (Naib 1984). Often there are scattered foci of infection located on the squamous and endocervical epithelia. Many biopsies will only reveal non-specific inflammatory changes (Josey et al. 1966).

Anus and Rectum

Goodell et al. (1983) biopsied 10 patients with herpetic proctitis. Non-specific changes noted in most included crypt abscesses, and infiltrates of polymorpho-nuclear leukocytes in the lamina propria. Multinuclear giant cells were only seen in a single biopsy specimen, although other specific changes including intranu-clear inclusions and an infiltration of lymphocytic cells around submucosal blood vessels were seen more frequently.

Lymph Nodes

The histological changes associated with herpetic lymphadenitis have been described by Lapsley et al. (1984). The basic architecture is distorted but preserved with marked hypercellularity and expansion of the paracortical areas. The cellular infiltrate consists largely of immunoblasts interspersed with lympho-cytes, plasmacytic cells and macrophages. The authors stressed the importance of not confusing the changes with those associated with malignancy. Similar changes have been described in association with Epstein–Barr virus infection (Salvador et al. 1971) and herpes zoster (Harstock 1968).

Severe Mucocutaneous and Disseminated HSV

Introduction

The clinical features of severe mucocutaneous and disseminated HSV are discussed in Chap. 5. The pathological features of severe mucocutaneous HSV

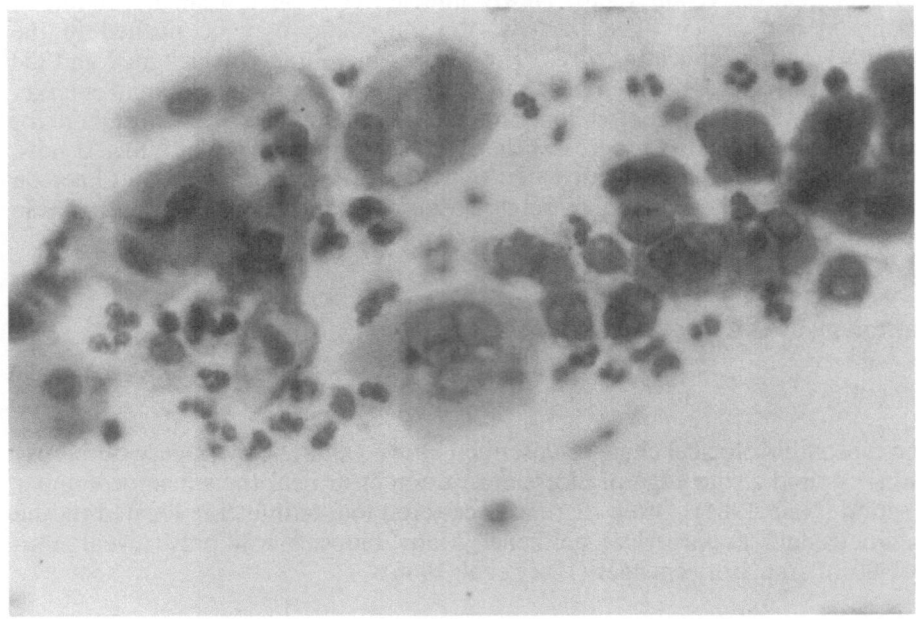

a

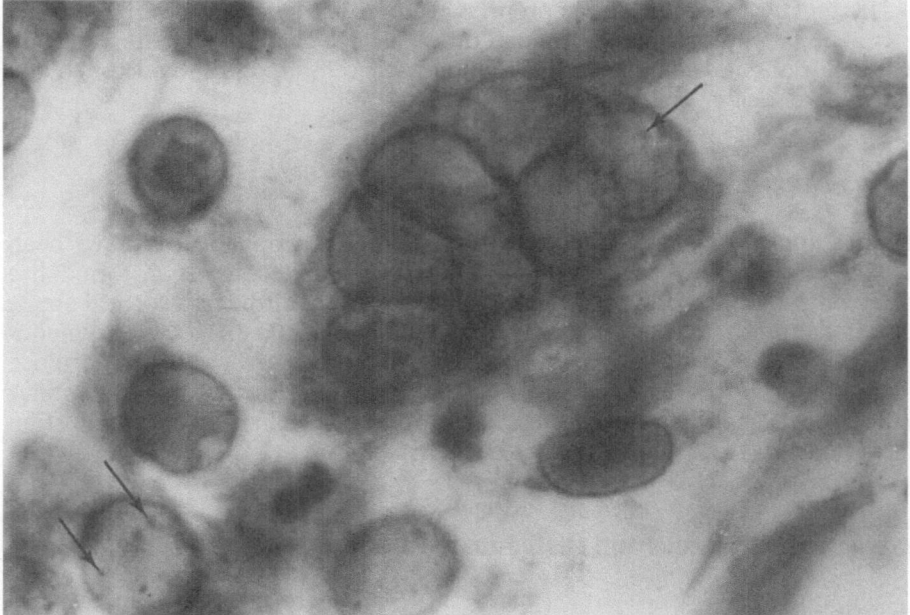

b

Fig. 6.2. a HSV cytology. Multi-nucleated giant cells and numerous polymorphonuclear leukocytes can be seen. **b** Multi-nucleated giant cells with numerous intranuclear inclusions. (**b** courtesy of Dr G Kocjan.)

are identical with the less severe infection (see above), except that larger areas of skin or mucous membranes are involved. When dissemination occurs (usually in immunocompromised patients), the virus may spread throughout the body. The organs commonly involved include the oesophagus, the lungs and the liver. Although HSV oesophagitis usually occurs in association with disseminated HSV, the condition has been described in isolation.

Herpetic Oesophagitis

Agha et al. (1986) have described three stages of mucosal damage associated with herpetic oesophagitis: (1) the presence of vesicles in the distal oesophagus; (2) coalescing of the vesicles into larger lesions (0.5–2 cm) with raised borders; (3) diffuse mucosal ulceration and necrosis. At endoscopy, herpetic lesions are described as "punched out" (Nash and Ross 1974), or "volcano" ulcers (Agha et al. 1986). The ulcers may be multiple or single, discreet or confluent, and localised or widespread.

Histologically typical giant cells with intranuclear inclusions can be found near the edge of ulcers or in sloughed squamous epithelium. Exfoliative cytology obtained by endoscopy may be an excellent way of making an early diagnosis (Lightdale et al. 1977).

Herpetic Hepatitis

Liver involvement with HSV carries a high mortality, and consequently most of the histological material has been obtained post mortem (Chase et al. 1987). McKenzie et al. (1959) described the pathological changes in the liver of eight malnourished children with disseminated herpes. In six of the eight cases there was a macroscopic appearance of the liver which the authors described as pathognomonic for herpes. The lesions consisted of circular foci of necrosis, white in colour and ranging from pinhead size to 3 mm. Each was surrounded by a zone of hyperaemia or haemorrhage. The lesions occurred throughout the liver parenchyma.

On microscopy, extensive destruction of hepatocytes is evident; at times the degree of destruction is so great that intact hepatocytes are only found in the periportal areas (Taylor et al. 1981). The necrotic areas are surrounded by haemorrhage but neither an inflammatory cell infiltrate nor a proliferation of liver cells occurs (Raga et al. 1984). Typical intranuclear inclusions may be seen (McKenzie et al. 1959; Raga et al. 1984; see Figs 6.3 and 6.4).

The cause of death is often disseminated intravascular coagulation and, at post mortem, widespread haemorrhagic areas (including the gastrointestinal tract, pleura, lung skin, mucous membranes) are seen. Herpetic involvement of other organs (including the lungs and brain) is not uncommon.

Infections of the Middle and Lower Respiratory Tract

Extensive herpetic ulceration of the middle and lower respiratory tract occurs in patients who have been extensively burned or those who have profound

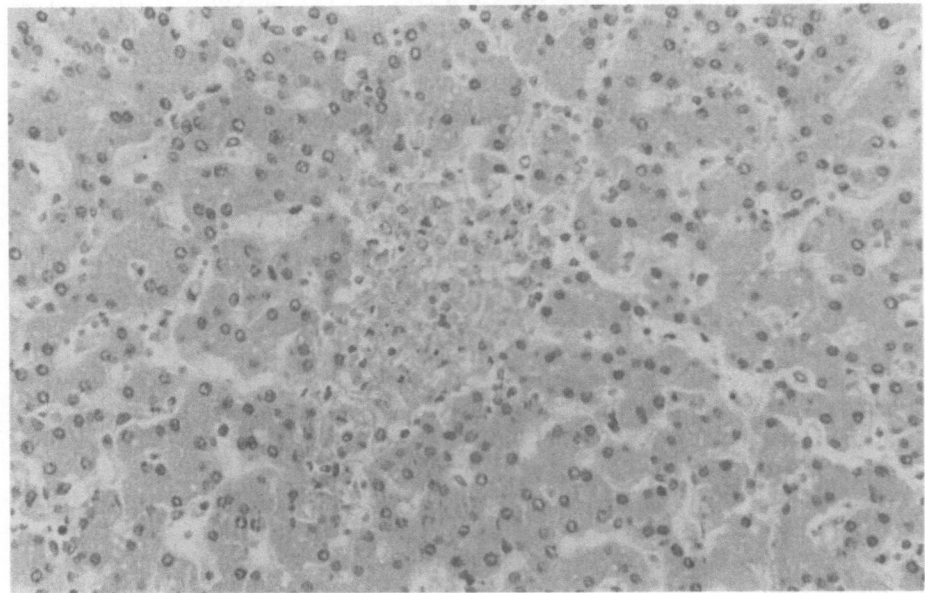

Fig. 6.3. Histopathology of HSV liver infection. Micro-abscess in the liver parenchyma, with destruction of liver tissue. Viral inclusions are evident. (Courtesy of Dr D Katz.) (× 90).

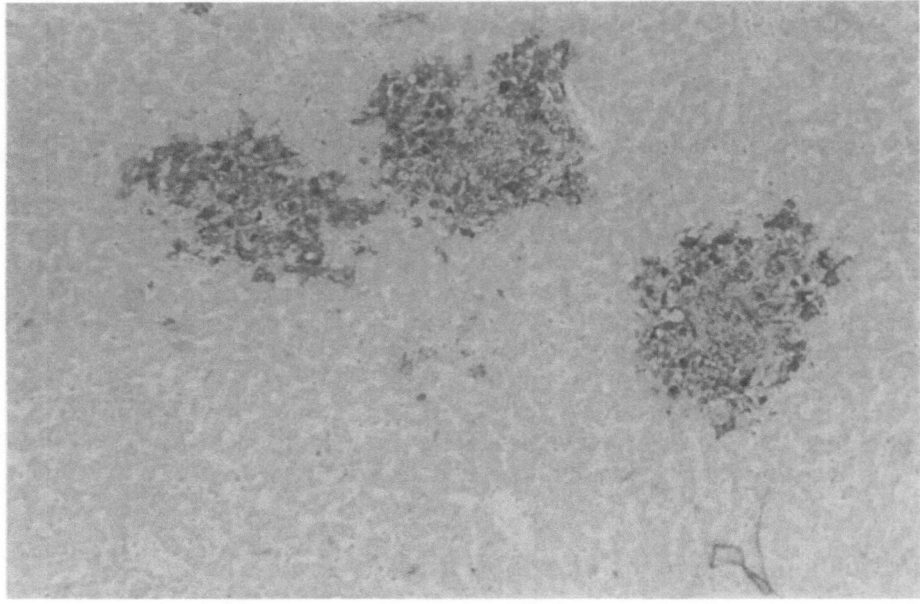

Fig. 6.4. Micro-abscess in liver stained with an immunoperoxide anti-HSV antibody. (Courtesy of Dr D Katz.) (× 90).

immunosuppression (see Chap. 5). Involvement of the trachea and larynx is a particular problem in burns patients who have been intubated (Nash and Foley 1970), whereas herpetic bronchopneumonia occurs in those who are immuno-compromised (Hull et al. 1984; Graham and Snell 1983). The histopathological features of lesions from the trachea, larynx and bronchi are similar. The epithelial surface shows extensive ulceration, with typical intranuclear inclusions and giant cells, and necrotic cells may be evident in the airway lumen. The surface of the ulcer may develop a membrane of fibrin, infiltrated with inflammatory cells, and necrotic epithelial cells (Nash and Foley 1970; Graham and Snell 1983).

The histological features of HSV pneumonitis are those of a necrotising bronchopneumonia. The gross appearance at autopsy is that of massive consoli-dation and haemorrhage. Microscopy shows sub-epithelial infiltration of the bronchi with mononuclear cells. The walls of the alveoli are necrotic and the alveoli themselves are filled with fibrin and necrotic debris. Occasional mono-nuclear cells may be seen. Haemorrhage may or may not be a feature. Typical intranuclear inclusions are usually evident in numerous bronchoepithelial cells (Douglas et al. 1969; Nash and Foley 1970; Hull et al. 1984).

Other Organs

Numerous other organs may be infected with HSV when the virus disseminates; these include the adrenal glands, spleen, stomach, intestines, pericardium, kidneys, pancreas, muscle and bone marrow (McKenzie et al. 1959; Raga et al. 1984; Walker et al. 1981).

Macroscopically the adrenal glands are usually normal but areas of necrosis may be seen microscopically in both the medulla and the cortex. Intranuclear inclusions may also be evident. The spleen is often enlarged and, as with the adrenals, areas of necrosis may be seen.

Occasionally HSV is isolated from other organs. Sometimes the organs appear normal and at other times areas of necrosis with or without intranuclear inclusions may be seen.

Encephalitis

HSV infection of the brain is often widespread but the virus does appear to have a predeliction for the temporal and frontal lobes. The lesions are often asymmetrical and the cortex is more involved than the white matter (Drachman and Adams 1962). Patients who have died often have supratentorial tissue which is softened and haemorrhagic. Histology of biopsy or post mortem tissue shows widespread cellular infiltration of the leptomeninges and perivascular spaces by lymphocytes and macrophages. Sometimes the macrophages form collections called macroglial nodules. In areas of extensive necrosis the neurones are shrunk with pyknic nuclei and typical eosinophilic intranuclear inclusions. The inclu-sions are usually seen in cortical nerve cells and oligodendrocytes (Fig. 6.5; see also McMenemey and Thomas Smith 1979; Anonymous 1979). The diagnosis of HSV encephalitis cannot always be made at the time of brain biopsy on

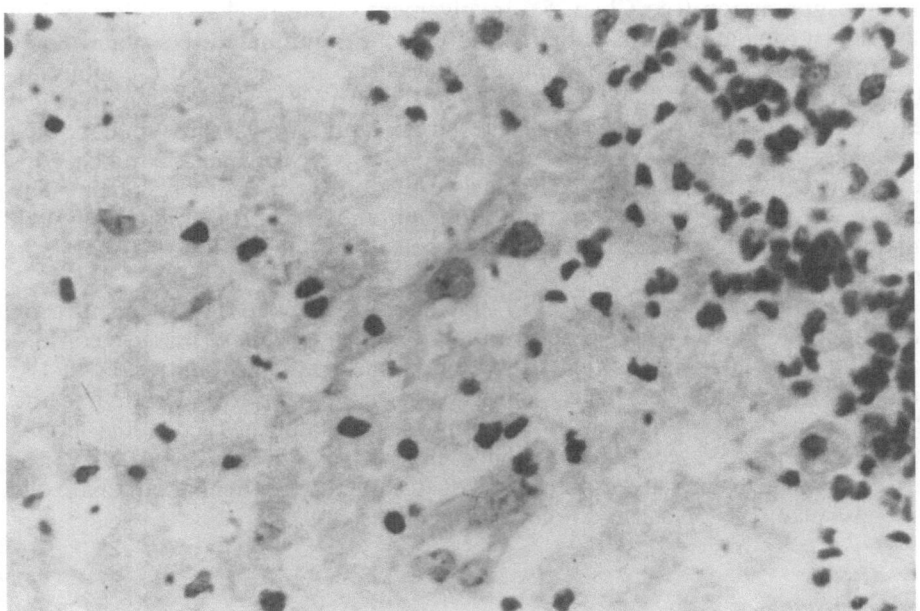

Fig. 6.5. HSV "encephalitis". Cellular infiltrate with lymphocytes and macrophages. Intranuclear inclusion in glial cells is evident. (Courtesy of Dr D Katz.) (× 300).

histological grounds alone. Other methods of detecting the virus may need to be used, including detection of HSV antigens, detection of viral DNA or visualisation of viral particles using electron microscopy. These various techniques are outlined in Chap. 7.

Meningitis and Radiculomyelopathy

The pathological features of these conditions are unknown.

Eye Infections

Virtually any part of the eye may be infected with HSV. The pathological features of HSV infection of the eyelid are identical with those occurring anywhere else on the skin. The features of conjunctivitis are not well documented, in contrast to HSV keratitis, where there have been several studies in humans and animals.

Dawson et al. in 1968 studied the histopathology of 19 corneal specimens from patients undergoing keratoplasty for chronic herpetic keratitis. The commonest findings were destruction of Bowman's membrane, cellular infiltration with polymorphonuclear leukocytes, lymphocytes and macrophages, and the presence of blood vessels in the stroma. Other changes included loss of the epithelial layer, increase in the basement membrane and production of connective tissue (pannus) between the epithelium and Bowman's membrane. In a few specimens, there was destruction of Descemet's membrane and formation of a dense retrocorneal membrane. Similar features have been described in experimentally infected animals (Wolter et al. 1956). The typical keratitic precipates consist of an infiltrate of macrophages, plasma cells, lymphocytes and fibrin (O'Connor 1976; Culbertson et al. 1982).

Any part of the uveal tract may be infected with HSV. The iris may be oedematous and infiltrated with a variety of inflammatory cells, including plasma cells, lymphocytes, eosinophils and macrophages; the ciliary body may have a similar infiltrate.

Choroidoretinitis occurs in neonates or those with severe immunosuppression (see Chap. 5). Many of these patients have keratoconjunctivitis, although others have no evidence of herpetic infection elsewhere in the eye (Nahmias and Hagler 1972). The choroid is thickened and infiltrated with plasma cells, and the sclera, episclera and ciliary bodies also have a heavy cellular infiltration with lymphocytes and plasma cells (Culbertson et al. 1982). Appearances within the retina may be varied with some areas totally necrotic, whereas in others there is focal necrosis with relatively normal retina between. Within the necrotic areas the architecture is destroyed and debris, red blood cells, macrophages and polymorphonuclear leukocytes may be seen. Some areas of necrosis may be close to retinal arteries. Where the architecture is preserved, scattered inflammatory cells may be seen and typical intranuclear inclusions visualised in the underlying pigment containing epithelial cells. The optic nerve may be necrotic and replaced by plasma cells and macrophages (Culbertson et al. 1982).

The histopathological features are similar to those seen with varicella zoster and cytomegalovirus infection (De Venecia et al. 1971; Schwartz et al. 1976).

Neonatal Herpes

Clinically, neonatal HSV is often divided into localised (to the skin, mouth or eyes – with or without central nervous system involvement) and disseminated. Whilst this is a very useful clinical and prognostic division, the pathological features are not different and depend only on the organs affected (Singer 1981).

The pathological features of neonatal cutaneous HSV are no different from those seen in adults (Singer 1981). Lesions on the skin may be very extensive and often occur initially on the presenting part (Nahmias et al. 1983). Lesions in the mouth are often more extensive than those seen in older children or adults. Infiltration of the underlying muscle with lymphocytes, monocytes and occasional neutrophils has also been described (Arje et al. 1955; Singer 1981).

The histological features of HSV oesophagitis and eye infection resemble those described in adults (Singer 1981; Hagler et al. 1969). Similarly the changes associated with neonatal herpetic hepatitis do not appear to be very different from those described in older children and adults with massive necrosis, haemorrhage and lack of inflammatory cell infiltrate (Hass 1935; Zueler and Stulberg 1952; Wright and Miller 1965; McDougal et al. 1954; Singer 1981).

In contrast, the pathology of central nervous system herpes in the neonate is different. In adults, the virus apears to have a predilection for the temporal and frontal lobes, whereas in the neonate the lesions are often more widely and diffusely spread in both the white and grey matter (Singer 1981). Lesions in the

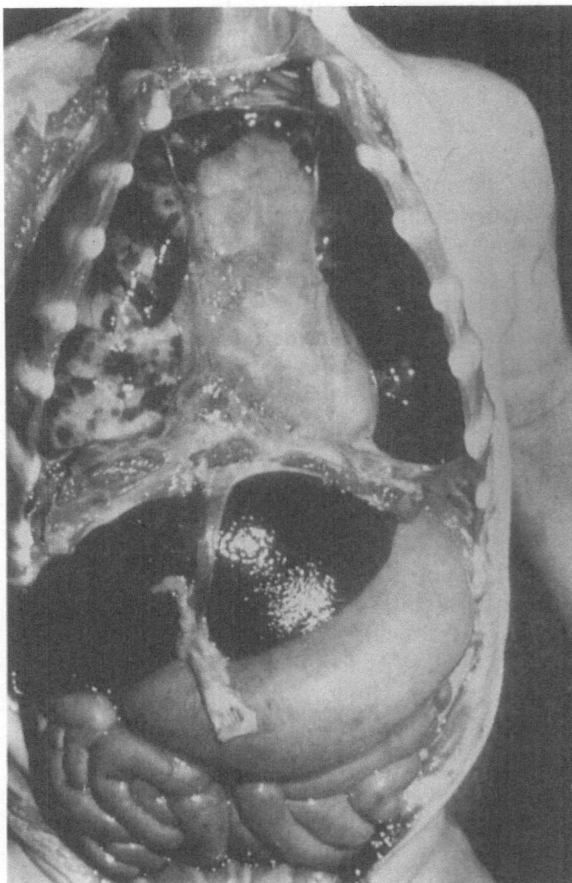

Fig. 6.6. Haemorrhagic areas in the lungs and liver due to disseminated intravascular coagulation in an infant with neonatal herpes post mortem.

brain stem and medulla are not uncommon (Zuelzer and Stulberg 1952; Singer 1981). A widespread cellular infiltration by lymphocytes and macrophage is usually seen around blood vessels, and typical inclusions may be seen in oligodendrocytes and cortical nerve cells.

Other organs, including the spleen, pancreas, lungs, ovary, muscle, heart and kidneys, are ocasionally infected (Nahmias et al. 1970; Arje et al. 1955; Singer 1981). The pathological features include areas of necrosis with or without typical inclusions.

The cause of death is often extensive central nervous system involvement; however, some neonates die as a result of bronchopneumonia or internal haemorrhage due to disseminated intravascular coagulation (Fig. 6.6).

The Placenta

There is a handful of reports of HSV infecting the placenta. In all these cases, foetal or neonatal herpes was an invariable association (Witzelben and Driscoll

1965; Altshuler 1974). The majority of cases of neonatal herpes are not diagnosed until several days after birth and it is therefore unknown how common placental involvement actually is. The pathological changes include areas of necrosis affecting groups of villi, usually with little inflammatory response (Witzelben and Driscoll 1965). Inclusion bodies may be seen.

Pathogenesis

Introduction

The pathogenesis of primary infection, latency and reactivation has been discussed at length in earlier chapters. The objectives of this section are to review the pathogenesis of some of the other aspects of herpetic infections, including symptomatic and asymptomatic viral excretion, various neurological problems, eye disease, neonatal herpes and the dissemination of HSV.

Symptomatic and Asymptomatic Viral Excretion

The majority of people who contract herpes do so from someone who is usually unaware that they are infected with the virus; and seroepidemiological surveys confirm that inapparent HSV infection is widespread (see Chap. 3). In addition, viral excretion from the genital tract or mouth in patients with no symptoms is also well documented (see Chap. 3). What determines when or whether symptoms and/or lesions develop is largely unknown. Several factors are suggested as triggers for symptomatic relapses; these include local trauma, exposure to ultraviolet light and menstruation, but whether these are also involved in asymptomatic viral excretion is unknown. One possible mechanism discussed at length in Chap. 2 is that viral reactivation occurs intermittently throughout the life of the individual in response to the normal physiological processes of renewal and repair, and that clinically apparent lesions occur only if there is mucosal damage at the time. This would seem to be a plausible explanation in those people who have clinical herpes from time to time but not in the vast number who never have obvious lesions. This argument should be countered with the observation that many patients with "asymptomatic herpes" when closely questioned or examined, do reveal clinical lesions suggestive of herpes (Mertz et al. 1985). Perhaps HSV is always shed from damaged mucosa; it is just that the lesions are not always obvious to the patient.

Neurological Problems

Viral Meningitis

Viral meningitis may occur in a small percentage of patients with a first attack of genital herpes (see Chap. 4). The illness is said to occur as a result of either a generalised viraemia, with haematogenous spread to the meninges (Craig and Nahmias 1973; Corey et al. 1983) or direct spread from mucosal surfaces via peripheral nerves (Overall et al. 1975). Although both these explanations are plausible, they do not explain why patients with severe primary gingivostomatitis do not develop meningitis. The answer may lie within the virus itself. Animal studies suggest that HSV 2 may be more neurovirulent than HSV 1 (McKendall 1980) and in addition it is possible that HSV 2 may be more capable of infecting peripheral nerves. The difference would then be explained on the basis that most genital infections are due to HSV 2 whilst most oral ones are due to HSV 1.

Radiculomyelopathy

Acute inflammatory radiculomyelopathy of the lumbrosacral region mainly affecting the sensory and autonomic nerves occurs in a small number of females with primary genital herpes and a considerable number of homosexual males with primary perianal and anal herpes (see Chap. 4). A similar syndrome occurs with varicella zoster infection of the sacral area (Jellinek and Tulloch 1976), due to inflammation of the sensory root ganglia (Denny-Brown et al. 1944). Examination of the cerebrospinal fluid in these patients reveals an increase in polymorphonuclear leukocytes, suggesting that an inflammatory response, possibly with oedema, is causing the problem. The extensive mucosal involvement associated with anal herpes and the probability that this may give rise to more heavily infected neurones may explain why homosexual men with anal herpes are more prone to this condition.

Encephalitis

There are two fascinating and as yet unanswered questions relating to HSV encephalitis. The first is "how does the virus reach the central nervous system?" and the second is "why does the virus have a predilection for the frontal and temporal lobes?"

It has been suggested that HSV tracks along the olfactory pathways to the frontal and nearby temporal lobes (Johnson and Mims 1968). Evidence supporting this view comes from studies where HSV has been detected in the olfactory tracts (Esiri 1982). If this is the explanation, how the virus gets into the olfactory nerves and what makes it migrate to the central nervous system remain unknown. Intranasal inoculation has been postulated (Johnson and Mims 1968) but why and how HSV is inoculated into the nose is unclear.

An alternative explanation is that HSV travels from its latent site in the trigeminal ganglia through the tentorial branches of the trigeminal nerve to the dura mater and then by direct cell-to-cell contact into the adjacent temporal and frontal cortices (Davis and Johnson 1979).

More recently a postulate was put forward by Damasio and van Hoesen (1985) based on the observation that HSV encephalitis is confined to limbic system. These authors suggest that HSV is transported from the trigeminal ganglion to the trigeminal nuclei. From there, via limbic-related nuclei such as the locus caeruleus and the raphe, the virus is transported to the cerebral cortices. Only in the limbic cortices (i.e. frontal and temporal) would it be able to multiply, with concomitant destruction of nerve cells. The major question unanswered by all three themes is "what makes a latent infection reactivate, move to a new site, and then cause widespread infection?"

"Neuralgia"

Recurrent "nerve pain", usually in the dermatomal distribution of the lesions, is a common and troublesome symptom for many patients with recurrent oral or genital herpes. It may occur prior to, or concurrent with the onset of the lesions (see Chap. 4). The most likely explanation for this phenomenon is non-specific neural stimulation at the time of viral reactivation – possibly explaining why the pain often precedes the lesions. Why these symptoms occur only in some patients and why in some they are the most troublesome aspect of the illness is unclear.

Dissemination

Dissemination of HSV infections from small, localised and well demarcated lesions to widespread cutaneous or visceral illness usually occurs as a result of depressed cell-mediated immunity (CMI) (see Chaps. 1 and 5). Recurrences are usually controlled and terminated by CMI responses. In patients with general depression of CMI, e.g. those with profound malnutrition, tumours, receiving chemotherapy or infection with human immunodeficiency virus (HIV), the recurrences become more severe, extend locally and may disseminate viscerally. In contrast, patients with problems of local immunity, in particular atopic eczema (Barker et al. 1988), the illness spreads widely and rapidly over the skin. Visceral involvement is not a common feature (Fig. 6.7).

There are two anomalies to this well-defined pattern. Firstly, only a minority of patients with depressed CMI disseminate viscerally, and, secondly, visceral dissemination occasionally occurs in patients who apparently have normal immunity (Chap. 5). Visceral dissemination may depend on a balance between the amount of virus in the circulation and the competence of the immune system at the time. Profound viraemia in the presence of a minimal depression in CMI (e.g. as a result of another viral infection) may explain oesophageal and/or hepatic involvement in people with apparently normal immunity.

Eye Infections

Most manifestations of HSV eye disease are due to direct damage caused by the virus itself, together with the inflammatory response (see Chap. 4). Dendritic ulcers probably occur as a result of a balance between epithelial destruction and repair, whereas with geographical ulcers there is more epithelial destruction (Dawson 1984). A number of aspects do not appear to be associated with active viral replication, including the occurrence of indolent ulcers and stromal keratitis. Indolent epithelial ulcers seldom contain live virus and appear to occur as a result of failure of re-attachment of the epithelium, corneal anaesthesia,

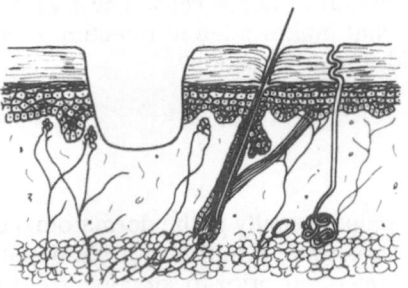

Normal immunity

Localised lesions on skin

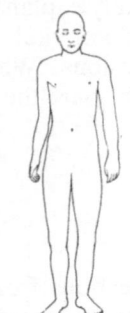

**Local depression of
cell-mediated immunity**

Widespread skin infection

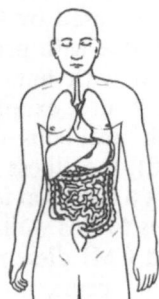

**General depression of
cell–mediated immunity**

Severe local infection +
disseminated internal infection

Fig. 6.7. The pathogenesis of *disseminated* HSV infection.

underlying stromal inflammation and the effects of drugs, in particular steroids
(Goldman et al. 1969; Dawson 1984).

The pathogenesis of stromal disease appears to be more complex. Live virus
does not survive in the avascular connective tissue of the stroma – but the
remaining viral proteins probably act as foreign bodies and are potent inducers
of antigen–antibody reactions (Rouse 1985). Two forms of immune reaction
have been described. One is antibody–antigen–complement mediated, and
presents as interstitial keratitis and limbal vasculitis (Meyers-Elliot et al. 1980);
the other is a delayed-type hypersensitivity reaction, where sensitised lymphocytes, plasma cells and even macrophages and polymorphonuclear leukocytes
invade the cornea, seeing various corneal elements as "foreign". (Dawson et al.
1968; Meyers and Chitjian 1976). The latter form of stromal illness is clinically
characterised by oedema and neovascularisation (see Chap. 4).

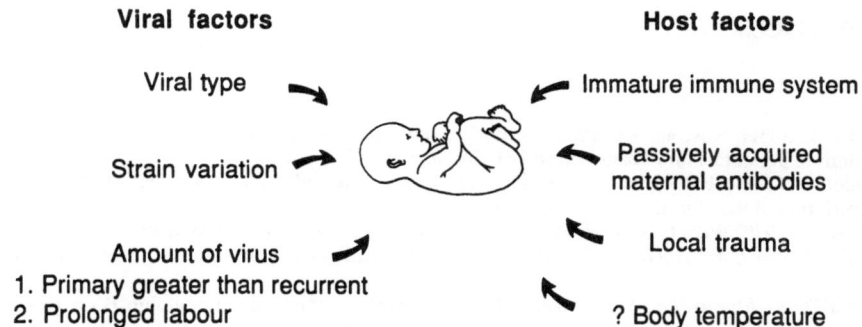

Fig. 6.8. The pathogenesis of a neonatal herpes, showing the relationship between *host* and *viral* *factors*.

Neonatal HSV

Neonatal herpes occurs when the newborn comes into contact with HSV, usually as a result of delivery through an infected birth canal. The reason why the virus disseminates in neonates is unclear. It has been suggested that non-specific defence mechanisms including natural killer cell and monocyte macrophage function may be less efficient in the new born (Mintz et al. 1980; Trofatter et al. 1979; Ching and Lopez 1979). The roles of T cells and immunoglobulins remain unknown.

Animal experiments suggest that body temperature may be important. In newborn puppies, who have a slightly lower body temperature for the first 3 weeks of life, a disseminated canine herpesvirus infection may occur (Carmichael et al. 1970). It is unknown whether minor temperature changes in human newborns are a factor.

The amount of virus to which the infant is exposed is also important. In primary genital herpes, viral titres are high and several sites (e.g. cervix, vulva and perineum) are usually involved (see Chap. 4). As a consequence, the newborn is invariably exposed to HSV often at high titre. In contrast, with recurrent genital herpes, viral titres are lower and the usual sites of involvement are external genitalia, perianal area, perineum or buttocks. Thus, contact with infected secretions is far less likely. The exposure time also is probably important, with prolonged labour increasing the risk.

The importance of passively acquired maternal antibodies has been discussed in Chap. 5. Although the importance of antibodies is disputed, it is likely that they confer partial protection.

Neonates with HSV 2 infection appear to have a worse neurological outcome than those with HSV 1 (Corey et al. 1988). It is unclear whether the difference is due to the virus itself or to the fact that some of the infants with HSV 1 probably acquired these infections from sources other than the birth canal, possibly suggesting a lower titre of virus and a shorter exposure to the virus (Bowman et al. 1988). It is evident that the pathogenesis of neonatal herpes is far from clear.

In summary, it is likely that the pathogenesis of neonatal infection is dependent upon several factors, including viral type, possible strain variation, immune factors, body temperature, maternal antibodies and the amount of virus to which the neonate is exposed (Fig. 6.8).

References

Agha FP, Lee HH, Nostrant TT (1986) Herpetic esophagitis: a diagnostic challenge in immunocompromised patients. Am J Gastroenterol 81: 246–253

Altshuler G (1974) Pathogenesis of congenital herpes virus infection. Case report including a description of the placenta. Am J Dis Child 127: 427–429

Anonymous (1979) Weekly clinicopathological conference case 44. N Engl J Med 301: 987–994

Arje SL, Austin CA, Sanchez AF (1955) Herpetic hepatitis of the newborn. Obstet Gynecol 6: 169–173

Barker JNWN, Algere VA, MacDonald DM (1988) Surface bound immunoglobin E on antigen-presenting cells in cutaneous tissue of atopic dermatitis. J Invest Dermatol 90: 117–121

Bowman CA, Woolley PD, Kinghorn GR (1988) Herpes simplex virus neonatal encephalitis. Lancet i: 646

Carmichael LE, Barnes FD, Percy DH (1970) Temperature as a factor in resistance of young puppies to canine herpesvirus. J Infect Dis 120: 669–678

Chase RA, Pottage JC, Haber MH, Kistler G, Jensen D, Levin S (1987) Herpes simplex viral hepatitis in adults: two case reports and review of the literature. Rev Infect Dis 9: 329–333

Ching C, Lopez C (1979) Natural killing of herpes simpex virus type 1-infected target cells. Normal human responses and influence of antiviral antibody. Infect Immun 26: 49–56

Corey L, Adams HG, Brown ZA, Holmes KK (1983) Genital herpes simplex virus infections: clinical manifestations, course and complications. Ann Intern Med 98: 958–972

Corey L, Whitley RJ, Stone EF, Mohan K (1988) Difference between herpes simplex virus type 1 and type 2 neonatal encephalitis in neurological outcome. Lancet i: 1–4

Cowdry EV (1934) The problem of intranuclear inclusions in viral disease. Arch Pathol Lab Med 18: 527–542

Craig C, Nahmias AJ (1973) Different patterns of neurologic involvement with herpes simplex virus types 1 and 2: isolation of herpes simplex virus type 2 from the buffy coat of 2 adults with meningitis. J Infect Dis 127: 365–372

Culbertson WW, Blumenkrantz MS, Haines H, Gass DM, Mitchell KB, Norton EWD (1982) The acute retinal necrosis syndrome. Ophthalmology 89: 1317–1325

Cunningham AL, Turner RR, Miller AC, Para MF, Merigan TC (1985) Evaluation of recurrent herpes simplex lesions – an immunohistological study. J Clin Invest 75: 226–233

Damasio AR, van Hoesen GW (1985) The limbic system and the localisation of herpes simplex encephalitis. J Neurol Neurosurg Psychiatry 48: 297–301

Davis LE, Johnson RT (1979) An explanation for the localisation of herpes simplex encephalitis. Ann Neurol 5: 2–5

Dawson CR (1984) Ocular herpes simplex virus infections. Clin Dermatol 2: 56–66

Dawson C, Togni B, Moore TE (1968) Structural changes in chronic herpetic keratitis: studied by light and electron microscopy. Arch Ophthalmol 79: 740–747

De Venecia G, Zu Rhein GM, Pratt MU, Kisken W (1971) Cytomegalic inclusion retinitis in an adult. A clinical histopathologic and ultrastructural study. Arch Ophthalmol 86: 44–57

Denny-Brown D, Adams RD, Fitzgerald PJ (1944) Pathologic features of herpes zoster: a note on "geniculate herpes". Arch Neurol 51: 216–231

Douglas RG, Anderson MS, Weg JG, et al. (1969) Herpes simplex virus pneumonia. JAMA 210: 902–904

Drachman DA, Adams RD (1962) Herpes simplex and acute inclusion-body encephalitis. Arch Neurol 7: 45–53

Esiri MM (1982) Herpes simplex encephalitis, an immunohistological study of the distribution of viral antigen within the brain. J Neurol Sci 54: 209–226

Goldman JN, Dohlman CH, Krovitt BA (1969) The basement membrane in recurrent epithelial erosion syndrome. Trans Am Acad Ophthalmol Otolaryngol: 73: 471–81

Goodell SE, Quinn TC, Mkrtichian E, Schuffler MD, Holmes KK, Corey L (1983) Herpes simplex virus proctitis and homosexual men: clinical, sigmoidoscopic and histopathological features. N Engl J Med 308: 868–871

Graham BS, Snell JD (1983) Herpes simplex virus infection of the adult lower respiratory tract. Medicine, Baltimore: 62: 384–393

Haber H, Milne JA, Symmers WSC (1980) The skin. In: Symmers WSC (ed) Systemic pathology, vol 6, 2nd edn. Churchill Livingstone, Edinburgh, pp 2626–2822

Hagler WS, Walters DV, Nahmias AJ (1969) Ocular involvement in neonatal herpes simplex virus infection. Arch Opthalmol: 82: 169–176

Harstock RJ (1968) Postvaccinal lymphadenitis. Hyperplasia of lymphoid tissue that simulates malignant lymphomas. Cancer 21: 632–649

Hass GM (1935) Hepato-adrenal necrosis with intranuclear inclusion bodies: report of a case. Am J Pathol 11: 127–142

Hull HF, Blumhager JD, Benjamin D, Corey L (1984) Herpes simplex viral pneumonitis in childhood. J Pediatr 104: 211–215

Jellinek EH, Tulloch WS (1976) Herpes zoster with dysfunction of bladder and anus. Lancet ii: 1219-1222

Johnson RT, Mims CA (1968) Pathogenesis of viral infections of the nervous system. N Engl J Med 278: 23–38, 84–92

Josey WE, Nahmias AJ, Naib ZM, Utley PM, McKenzie WJ, Coleman MT (1966) Genital herpes simplex infection in the female. Am J Obstet Gynecol: 96, 493–501

Lapsley M, Kettle P, Sloan JM (1984) Herpes simplex lymphadenitis: a case report and review of the published work. J Clin Pathol 37: 1119–1122

Lightdale CJ, Wolf DJ, Marcucci RA, et al. (1977) Herpetic esophagitis in patients with cancer: antemortem diagnosis by brush cytology. Cancer 39: 223–226

McDougal RA, Beamer PR, Hellerstein S (1954) Fatal herpes simplex hepatitis in a newborn infant. Am J Clin Pathol 24: 1250–1258

McKendall RR (1980) Comparative neurovirulence and latency of HSV 1 and HSV 2 following foot pad inoculation in mice. J Med Virol 5: 25–32

McKenzie D, Hansen JDL, Becker W (1959) Herpes simplex virus infection: dissemination in association with malnutrition. Arch Dis Child 34: 250–256

McMenemey WH, Thomas Smith W (1979) The central nervous system. In: Symmers WSC (ed) Systemic pathology, vol 5, 2nd edn. Churchill Livingstone, Edinburgh, pp 2041–2159

Mertz GJ, Schmidt O, Jourden JL et al. (1985) Frequency of acquisition of first episode genital infection with herpes simplex virus from symptomatic and asymptomatic source contacts. Sex Transm Dis 12: 33–39

Meyers R, Chitjian P (1976) Immunology of herpes virus infection: immunity to herpes simplex virus in eye infections. Surv Ophthalmol 21: 194–204

Meyers-Elliot R, Pettit R, Maxwell W (1980) Viral antigens in the immune rings of herpes simplex stromal keratitis. Arch Ophthalmol 98: 897–904

Mintz H, Drew WL, Hoo R, Finley TN (1980) Age dependent resistance of human alveolar macrophages to herpes simplex virus. Infect Immun 28: 417–420

Nahmias AJ, Hagler WS (1972) Ocular manifestations of herpes simplex in the newborn (neonatal ocular herpes). Int Ophthalmol Clin 12: 191–213

Nahmias AJ, Alford CA, Korones SB (1970) Infection of the newborn with herpes virus hominis. Adv Paediatr 17: 185–226

Nahmias AJ, Keyserling HH, Kerríck G (1983) Herpes simplex. In: Remington J S, Klein J O (eds) Infectious diseases of the fetus and newborn infant. Saunders WB, Philadelphia, pp 156–190

Naib ZM (1966) Exfoliative cytology of viral cervico-vaginitis. Acta Cytol (Baltimore) 10: 126–129

Naib ZM (1984) Cytologic diagnosis of herpes simplex virus infection. Clin Dermatol 2: 83–89

Nash G, Foley FD (1970) Herpetic infection of the middle and lower respiratory tract. Am J Clin Pathol 54: 857–863

Nash G, Ross JS (1974) Herpetic esophagitis, a common cause of esophageal ulceration. Hum Pathol 5: 339–345

O'Connor GR (1976) Recurrent herpes simplex uveitis in humans. Surv Ophthalmol: 21, 165–170

Overall JC, Kern ER, Schlitzer RL, Friedman SB, Glasgow LA (1975) Central herpesvirus hominis infection in mice. I. Development of an experimental model. Infect Immun 11: 476–480

Raga J, Chrystal V, Coovadia HM (1984) Usefulness of clinical features and liver biopsy in diagnosis of disseminated herpes simplex infection. Arch Dis Child 59: 820–824

Rouse BT (1985) Immunopathology of herpesvirus infection. In: Roizman B, Lopez C (eds) The herpesviruses: immunobiology and prophylaxis of human herpesvirus infection, vol 4. Plenum Press, New York, pp 103–119

Salvador AN, Harrison EG, Kyle RA (1971) Lymphadenopathy due to infectious mononucleosis. Its confusion with malignant lymphoma. Cancer 27: 1029–1040

Schwartz JN, Cashwell F, Hawkins HK, Klintworth GK (1976) Necrotizing retinopathy with herpes zoster opthalmicus: a light and electron microscopical study. Arch Pathol Lab Med 100: 386–391

Singer DB (1981) Pathology of neonatal herpes simplex virus infections. In: Rosenberg HS, Berstein J (eds) Perspectives in pediatric pathology, vol 6, Masson, New York, pp 243–278

Taylor RJ, Saul SH, Dowling JN, Hakala TR, Peel RL, Ho M (1981) Primary disseminated herpes
    simplex infection with fulminant hepatitis following renal transplantation. Arch Intern Med 141:
    1519–1521
Trofatter KF Jr, Daniels CA, Williams RJ Jr, Gall SA (1979) Growth of type 2 herpes simplex virus
    in newborn and adult mononuclear leukocytes. Intervirology 11: 117–123
Walker DP, Longson M, Lawler W, Mallick NP, Davies JS, Johnson RWG (1981) Disseminated
    herpes simplex virus infection with hepatitis in an adult renal transplant recipient. J Clin Pathol
    34: 1044–1046
Witzelben CL, Driscoll SG (1965) Possible transplacental transmission of herpes simplex infection.
    Pediatrics 36: 192–199
Wolter JR, Shapiro I, Whitehouse F (1956) Pathology of experimental primary herpetic keratitis in
    rabbits. J Ophthalmol 41: 639–645
Wright HT Jr, Miller A (1965) Fatal infection in a newborn infant due to herpes simplex viruses.
    Report of a case diagnosed before death. J Pediatr 67: 130–132
Zuelzer WW, Stulberg CS (1952) Herpes simplex virus as the cause of fulminating visceral disease
    and hepatitis in infancy. Report of eight cases and isolation of the virus in one case. Am J Dis
    Child 83: 421–439

Chapter 7

Laboratory Diagnosis

Introduction

The cultivation of HSV from infected secretions or tissues is the most widely used and most sensitive technique for the diagnosis of herpes simplex infection. Other techniques which may be used include the detection of viral particles or viral antigens in infected tissues, histopathological features consistent with HSV on biopsy, and the use of serological tests. The sensitivity of most of these techniques depends on the amount of virus in the specimen. This in turn is dependent on lesion stage (vesicles and ulcers contain more virus than crusts), whether the attack is primary or recurrent (more virus in the primary attack) and on the immune status of the patient (immunosuppressed patients generally have more virus).

Viral Isolation in Cell Culture

The standard laboratory technique for detecting HSV is by isolation of the virus in tissue culture. For this purpose live intact virus needs to be transported to the laboratory in a suitable transport medium such as Hank's balanced salt solution with antibiotics, or veal infusion broth. Suitable material for culture includes vesicle fluid or cells from the base of ulcers (Table 7.1; see also Hsiung et al. 1984a). Faulty specimen-taking techniques (e.g. failure to remove the roof of the vesicles or insufficiently vigorous scraping from ulcers) probably account for a considerable number of false negative results. Specimens should be transported to the laboratory as soon as possible. If a delay of several hours is expected, specimens can be stored in a refrigerator at 4 °C. Biopsy or autopsy material is also suitable for culture. It should be minced and then a 10% (w/v) tissue suspension inoculated directly into the cell culture system.

Table 7.1 Specimens for HSV culture

Clinical problem	Specimen
Orolabial herpes	Vesicle fluid, material from base of ulcers
Genital herpes	Vesicle fluid, material from base of ulcers
Eye infection	Swabs or scrapes from ulcers, biopsy material
Encephalitis	Brain biopsy, temporal lobe
Disseminated visceral infection	
Oesophagitis	Swabs from ulcers or washings
Liver	Liver biopsy
Lung	Bronchoalveolar lavage, Transbronchial biopsy, open lung biopsy
Neonatal herpes	Vesicle fluid, material from base of ulcers or denuded skin
	Liver biopsy
	? Other tissue (as above)

HSV may be cultured in a variety of cell lines, including human diploid fibroblast lines such as human embryonic tonsil (HET), embryonic lung (HEL), embryonic kidney (HEK) or human amnion cells, and various animal cells including rabbit kidney (RK), African green monkey kidney (VERO), baby hamster kidney (GBK) or Guinea pig embryo (GPE) cells (Hsiung et al. 1984b; McSwiggan et al. 1975).

HSV produces a typical cytopathic effect (CPE) commencing as rounding of cells, which eventually become swollen, refractile and ultimately die and detach from the surface of the culture plate or well (Fig. 7.1). CPE can be seen as early as 12 h or as late as 7 days after inoculation (Herrmann and Stewart 1981).

HSV may be confirmed using a simple neutralisation test. This relies on the ability of viral antibodies to combine with virus and render it non-infectious. Reduction of plaques or inhibition of CPE is the most widely used (Zheng et al. 1983). More rapid techniques for identification of isolates include the use of immunofluorescence (Schmidt et al. 1980) or immunoperoxidase (Benjamin 1977) tests.

Typing of Isolates

Typing of HSV isolates is not performed routinely in many laboratories; however, it has a number of important uses. Firstly, it may help in predicting the likely outcome in patients with genital herpes and may help in counselling (see Chap. 4). Secondly, it may have application in epidemiological studies (see Chap. 3). Finally, with the introduction of new antiviral drugs, typing may help in deciding optimum therapy (see Chap. 8).

There are a number of biological differences between HSV 1 and HSV 2 which can be used in typing isolates. Firstly, HSV 1 grows poorly, whereas HSV 2 grows well, in primary chick embryo fibroblast culture (Figuero and Rawls 1969). Secondly, HSV 1 produces small pocks, and HSV 2 large pocks, on chorionic membranes of embryonated hens eggs (Nahmias and Dowdle 1968). Thirdly, low concentrations of deoxynucleosides such as thymidine markedly

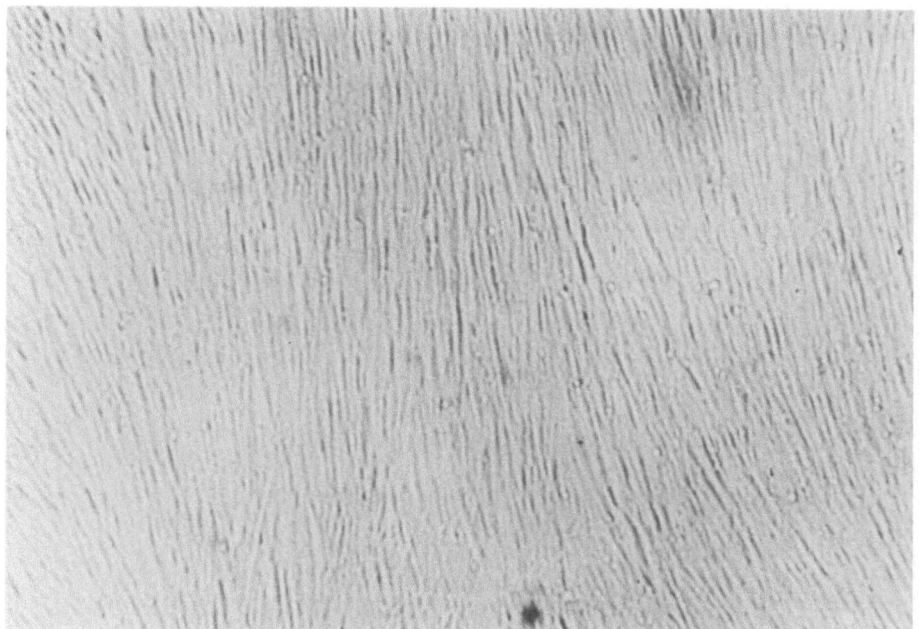

Fig. 7.1. Cytopathic effect (CPE) **a** Uninfected cell culture.

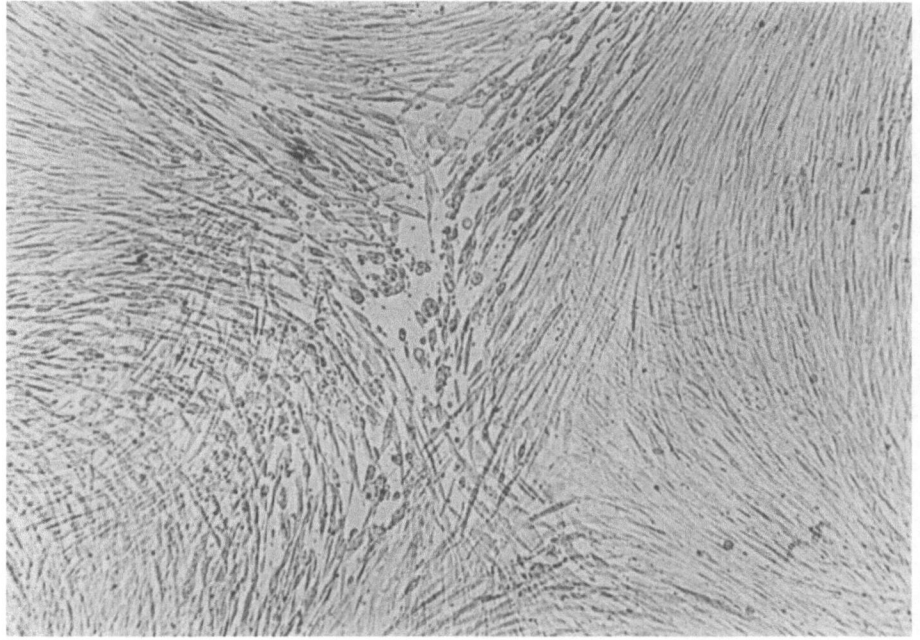

Fig. 7.1. (*continued*) **b** Early CPE: a few cells beginning to die and become round.

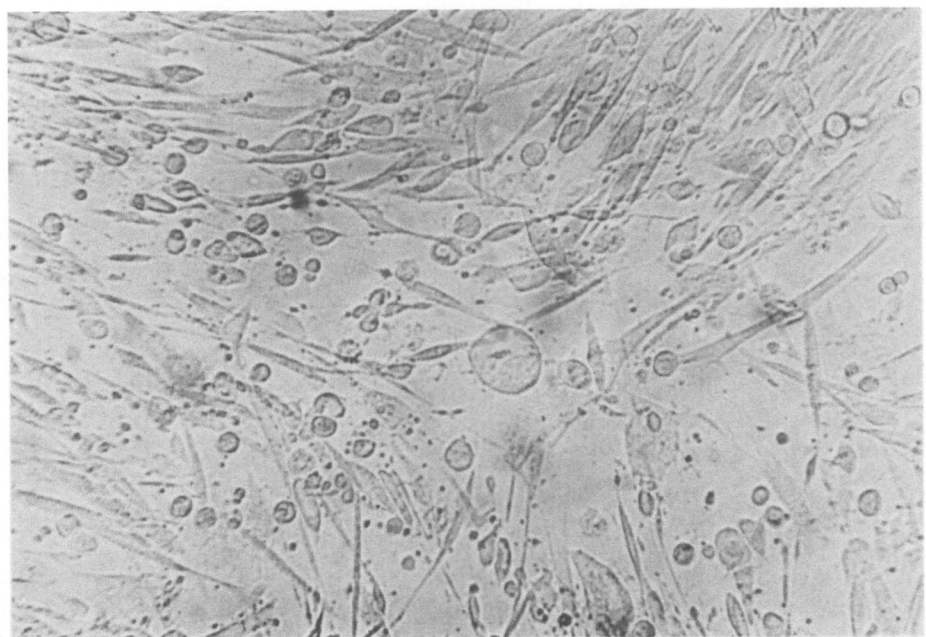

c

Fig. 7.1. (*continued*) **c** Moderate CPE: the majority of the cells rounding up and detaching from the surface.

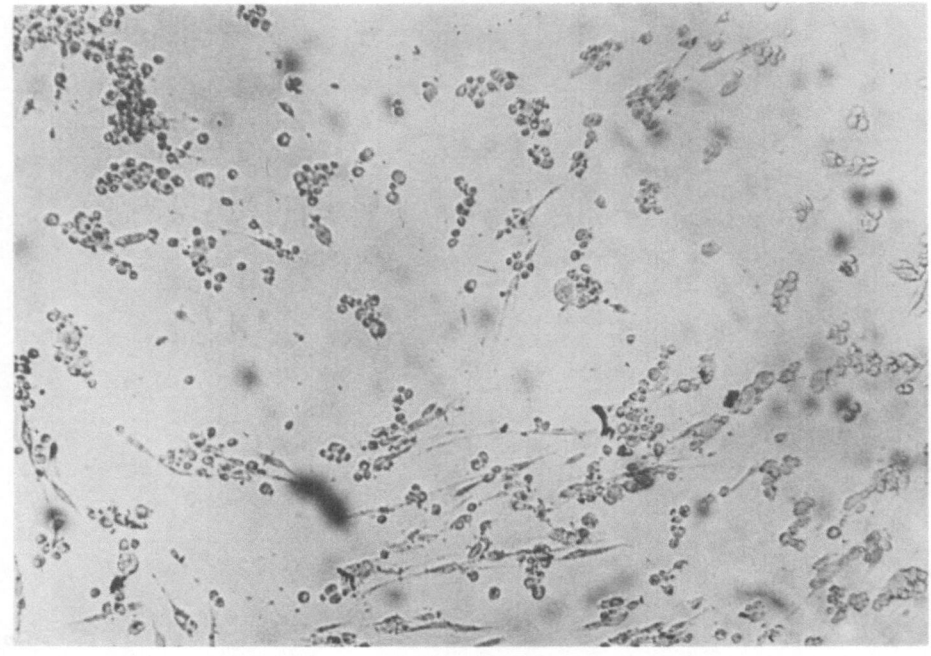

d

Fig. 7.1. (*continued*) **d** Late CPE: no live cells. (**a–d** Courtesy of Dr G Patou.)

inhibit the production of CPE in cell lines infected with HSV 2, whereas those infected with HSV 1 show no such inhibition (Kelman et al. 1975).

A number of immunological techniques have also been employed for differentiation between the two viral types. These tests all rely on the fact that the reaction is more intense with the homologous than with the heterologous antiserum, and all are limited by the considerable cross-reactivity between HSV 1 and HSV 2. Tests which have been used include an indirect immunoperoxidase test (Benjamin 1977), a direct immunofluorescence test (Nahmias et al. 1969), an enzyme-linked immunosorbent assay (ELISA) (Vestergaard and Grauballe 1979) and an indirect haemaglutination test (Bernstein and Stewart 1971). The introduction of monoclonal antibodies to HSV subtypes has vastly improved the sensitivity and specificity of these tests (Chan 1983; Sutherland et al. 1986), which are now widely available, reliable and relatively simple.

The recent introduction of restriction enzyme technology has opened the way not only for the unambiguous differentation of HSV 1 and 2, but also, for "fingerprinting" individual strains (Lonsdale 1979). This technique relies on cleavage of the double-stranded DNA at specific nucleotide sequences by certain restriction endonucleases (a type of bacterial enzyme) to produce fragments, the electrophoretic pattern of which is highly characteristic for that DNA. This technique has been used to demonstrate the uniqueness of HSV isolates from different individuals (Lonsdale et al. 1980), to document separate isolates from the same individual (Fife et al. 1983; Mindel and Sutherland 1983) and to identify and chart the cause of common source outbreaks (Fig. 7.2; see also Buchman et al. 1978).

Rapid Diagnostic Tests (Table 7.2)

The rapid confirmation of clinically suspected or asymptomatic HSV infections may be very important in several clinical settings. It will allow the early use of antiviral drugs in patients with life-threatening disseminated or neonatal herpes and will also improve the ability of the obstretician to make a rational decision regarding the management of maternal HSV infection detected at the time of

Table 7.2. Rapid diagnostic tests for HSV

Test	Comments
Tzanck test or Pap smear	Rapid. Poor sensitivity/specificity
EM	Rapid. Needs special equipment. Poor sensitivity/specifity
Antigen detection to speed cell culture (immunofluorescence, immunoperoxidase, ELISA)	Take 8–24 h, false negative if viral titres low. Cost effective
Antigen detection from direct smears Immunofluorescence or ELISA with monoclonal antibodies	Good sensitivity and specificity. Still being evaluated. Poor for cervical smears
DNA hybridisation	Technically difficult. Not suitable for widespread use

Pap., Papanicolau; EM, electron microscopy; ELISA, enzyme-linked immunosorbent assay.

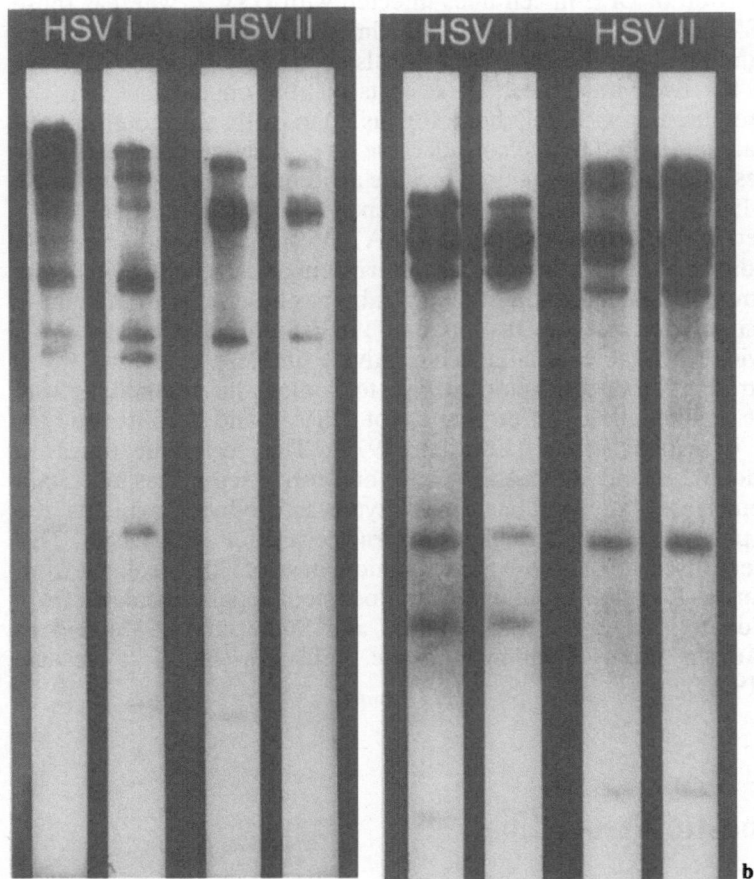

Fig. 7.2. Restriction enzyme technology for typing isolates.
a Electrophoretic patterns of *HSV 1* and *HSV 2* following digestion of *Hind*III restriction endonuclease. **b** Electrophoretic pattern of *HSV 1* and *HSV 2* following digestion of *Eco*RI endonuclease.

delivery (see Chap. 8). Since the introduction of effective non-toxic antiherpetic therapy, the pressure for early laboratory confirmation of suspected HSV infection is no longer such an important issue, as clinicians are willing to commence therapy pending the results of viral cultures.

Cytology and Electron Microscopy

The simplest method of rapidly diagnosing HSV infection is cytologically. Unna (1883) described the cellular changes associated with herpes virus infection: namely, multinuclear giant cells with eosinophilic intranuclear inclusions. These cytological findings are the basis for the Tzanck test and detection of HSV on Papanicolau smears. To do the Tzanck test, the lesion is scraped, smears made,

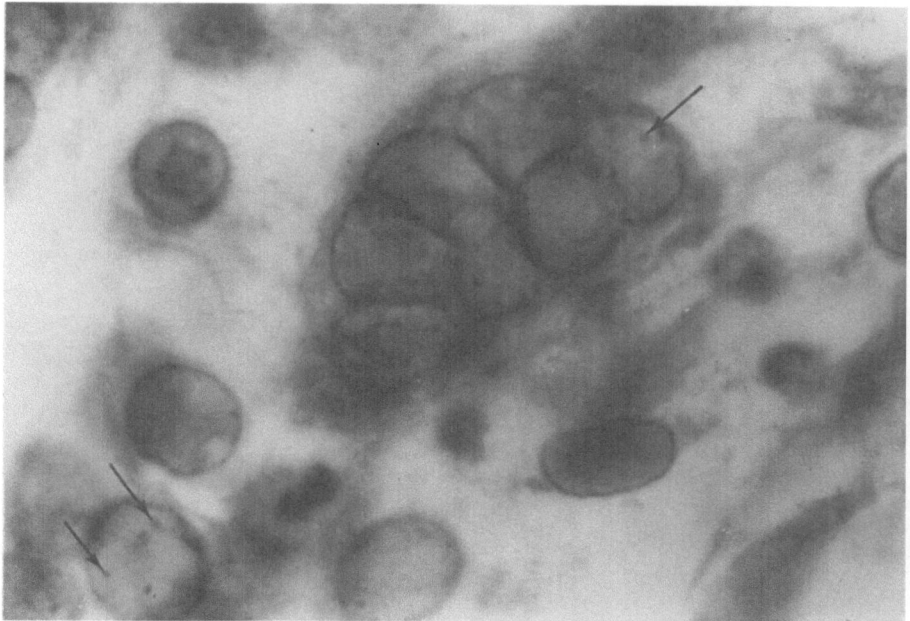

Fig. 7.3. HSV cytology. Multinucleated giant cells, and intranuclear inclusions. (Courtesy of Dr G Kocjan).

fixed and stained with Giemsa or Wright's stain, and the multinucleated giant cells detected by microscopy (see Fig. 7.3; see also Naib 1966). The test is quick but unfortunately insensitive, detecting, for example, only 40% of genital infections (Corey 1982). It also will not distinguish between HSV and varicella zoster (Naib 1984).

Herpes group viruses may be identified by direct examination of clinical specimens by electron miscroscopy (EM) after negative staining (Fig. 7.4). This technique has several limitations: firstly, specialised equipment is required; secondly, EM does not differentiate between HSV and other members of the herpes virus group (varicella zoster, cytomegalovirus, and Epstein–Barr virus); finally sensitivity is poor (Brown et al. 1979).

Antigen Detection

A number of methods have been developed for the rapid detection of HSV antigens, either to test clinical specimens directly or to enhance the sensitivity and speed of diagnosis by conventional cell culture. The tests involve the use of polyclonal or monoclonal antibodies in immunological assays including immuno-fluorescence (IF), immunoperoxidase (IP), and ELISA.

Detection of HSV antigens from direct clinical specimens is potentially the most rapid, reliable and reproducible method for the early detection of HSV

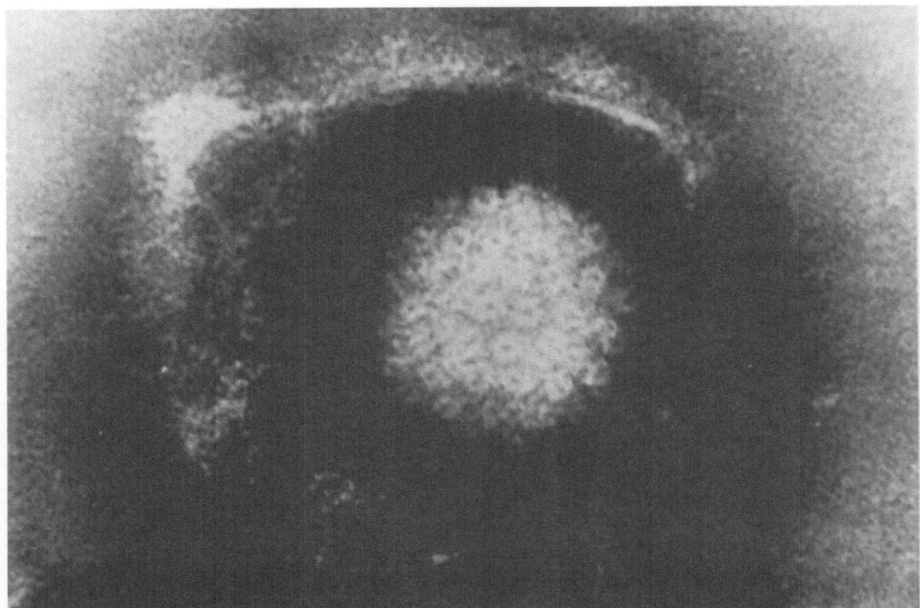

Fig. 7.4. Electron microscopy of HSV, using negative stain, showing the envelope and icosahedral nuclear capsid.

infection. Early results with indirect immunoperoxidase and direct immuno-fluorescence using polyclonal antibodies were disappointing, with a considerable percentage of false positive and negative results (Benjamin 1977; Mosely et al. 1981). The use of monoclonal antibodies has improved the sensitivity of the direct IF test and has the added advantage of typing the virus (Lafferty et al. 1987; Sutherland et al. 1986). A recent study from Seattle, WA (Lafferty et al. 1987), in patients with recurrent genital herpes showed that IF apparently detected more positive cases than viral cultures. In an attempt to determine whether these were false positive results, the authors followed up the cases for 6 months and were able to culture virus of the same type in 82% of their patients. False negative results, particularly from cervical specimens, unfortunately remain a problem.

The disadvantage of direct IF is that it requires a skilled microscopist, thus limiting the number of specimens that can be processed. Automated tests to detect HSV antigen, including ELISA (Grillner and Landquist 1983; Land et al. 1984; Lawrence et al. 1984; Morgan and Smith 1984; Nerurkar et al. 1983; Clayton et al. 1986) and radio immunoassay (RIA) (Forghani et al. 1974) have been developed. A recently evaluated ELISA using enzyme amplification and monoclonal antibodies showed that the sensitivity and specificity of this test was considerably greater than conventional ELISA techniques (Clayton et al. 1986). Although the test was highly specific, a small number of specimens which were positively identified by cell culture were negative on ELISA. This test may well offer an alternative to cell culture, as it is rapid, can be automated and requires little in the way of special expertise.

The use of IF tests with monoclonal antibodies may have other interesting applications. We recently evaluated such a test (Sutherland et al. 1986). Using a panel of 12 selected monoclonal antibodies we were able to identify seven different and distinct patterns of IF, from isolates of patients with primary genital herpes. These patients were followed for 6 months and subsequent recurrences also assessed. Of the 12 patients with HSV 2, 11 had recurrences and in 7 patients these were of the same subtype. However, in the remaining four patients some of the recurrences were different, suggesting either that the variation may be due to adaption in a new host or that the patient may have been "reinfected". This test may prove to be a useful adjunct to endonuclease restriction analysis for epidemiological studies of herpes infections. A recently developed technique using a biotin-linked anti-HSV antibody and an avidin-fluorescein conjugate was said to be more specific by reducing Fc receptor binding to the Fc portion of the antibody (Nerurkar et al. 1983). The biotin-linked antibody binds very efficiently to avidin. This is readily detected following the addition of fluorescein-labelled avidin antibodies.

One of the methods used to speed up the diagnosis is to detect viral antigens in short-term cell cultures. These tests detect antigen 8–24 h after the clinical specimen has been inoculated into cell culture (anywhere from 24–72 h before CPE is evident), are 90%–95% as sensitive as cell culture, and are claimed to be cost effective. False negatives occur in specimens with low titres of HSV, and false positive results arising from toxicity in the tissue culture have been described (Corey 1986). Several tests have been developed including IF and IP tests and ELISA (Rubin and Rogers 1984; Salmon et al. 1984; Johnson et al. 1985; Mayo et al. 1985; Shekarchi et al. 1985).

The methods using monoclonal (as opposed to polyclonal antibodies) have the advantage of typing the isolate at the same time as the antigen is detected (Peterson et al. 1983; Goldstein et al. 1983; Gleaves et al. 1985; Frame et al. 1985).

DNA Hybridisation

There are two basic techniques for the detection of viral genomes by hybridisation of virus-specific probes to nucleic acids. In one, fragments of viral DNA which have been extracted from infected tissue can be detected using an identical, or partially identical, viral DNA which has been previously isolated, purified and labelled either with a radioisotope or with biotin. This is called DNA–DNA hybridisation or hybridisation in vitro (Fig. 7.5; see also Maniatis et al. 1982; Minson and Darby 1982; Meinkoth and Wahl 1984). The other technique is hybridisation in situ, using tissue sections rather than extracted DNA (Haase et al. 1984).

DNA probes may be useful in the development of techniques for HSV diagnosis and also for understanding the pathogenesis of HSV infections. However, they are not as yet sufficiently simple or automated for widespread use. In one study, the detection of HSV DNA from genital secretions using an HSV 1 probe was shown to be dependent on the number of copies of target

Biopsy DNA   Labelled HSV probe DNA

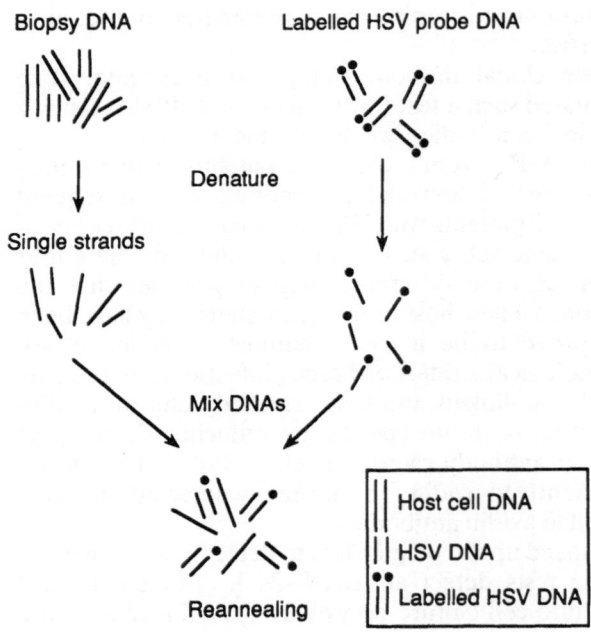

Fig. 7.5. *DNA–DNA* hybridisation in vitro. *Biopsy DNA* is denatured and mixed with *labelled HSV probe*. *Reannealing* occurs, allowing detection of the *labelled HSV*.

DNA. When the HSV 1 probe was used to detect HSV 2 the sensitivity was markedly reduced. In addition, the HSV 1 probe had a 90% sensitivity compared to viral culture for the detection of HSV 1 eye infection in rabbits (Redfield et al. 1983).

The research applications of these methods are numerous and the technique has already been used to try to unravel the complex issues of latency and oncogenesis (see Chap. 2). Indeed, radioisotopically labelled probes have been used to detect HSV 1 in brain and other neuronal tissues in human and experimentally infected mice (Sequiera et al. 1979; Galloway et al. 1979; Cabrera et al. 1980; Fraser et al. 1981) and HSV 2 from cervical carcinoma tissues

Serology

The serological diagnosis of HSV infection is complicated by the diversity of available assays, the extensive antigenic cross-reactivity between HSV 1 and HSV 2, because only 5% of patients with recurrent mucocutaneous infections produce a four-fold rise in antibody titre, and finally because the presence of IgM antibody to HSV reflects an active herpetic infection not necessarily a primary one. Serological tests have little value in the diagnosis and management of HSV infections. Many methods have been used to detect HSV antibodies in serum, including neutralisation, complement fixation, ELISA, RIA, passive and indirect haemoglobulin and immunoprecipitation.

Studies using polyvalent sera and monoclonal antibodies have shown that type-common antigenic determinants are shared by the majority of glycoproteins specified by the two herpes viruses (Pereira et al. 1980). However, glycoprotein G does appear to be type specific. Assays using purified glyco-protein prepared with monoclonal antibodies to type-specific HSV 1 and HSV 2 glycoprotein G, designated gG1 and gG2, have been developed. Lee et al. (1985, 1986) have developed an immunodot enzymic assay and Ashley et al. (1988) a modified Western blot technique.

These tests appear to be more specific, sensitive and reproducible than all previous serological assays. However, larger studies, particularly from individuals known to be infected with both types, remain to be done to establish their value finally.

Type-specific serological assays will be extremely useful in epidemiological and natural history studies and in the diagnosis and management of asymptomatic contacts of patients with clinical herpes. These tests may also prove helpful in the diagnosis and prevention of neonatal herpes by identifying "at risk" mothers in pregnancy (see Chap. 8).

Conclusions

In clinical medicine, cell culture remains the "gold standard" for the detection of HSV, although some of the newer techniques to detect HSV antigens using monoclonal antibodies may well offer a suitable alternative.

Serological tests (including the new type-specific ones) have a limited clinical application, but are already proving very useful for epidemiological studies.

The use of DNA hybridisation and restriction endonuclease analysis is at present limited to research into the epidemiology, pathogenesis and potential oncogenesis of HSV infections.

References

Ashley R, Militoni J, Lee F, Nahmias A, Corey L (1988) Comparison of Western blot (immunoblot) and glycoprotein G specific immunodot enzyme assay for detecting antibodies to herpes simplex virus types 1 and 2 in human sera. J Clin Microbiol 26: 662–667

Benjamin DR (1977) Use of immunoperoxidase for rapid diagnosis of mucocutaneous herpes simplex virus infection. J Clin Microbiol 6: 511–573

Bernstein MT, Stewart JA (1971) Method for typing antisera to herpesvirus hominis by indirect haemagglutination inhibition. Appl Microbiol 21: 680–684

Brown ST, Jaffe HW, Zaidi A, et al. (1979) Sensitivity and specificity of diagnostic tests for genital infection with herpes virus hominis. Sex Transm Dis 6: 10–13

Buchman TG, Roizman B, Adams G, Stover BH (1978) Restriction endonuclease fingerprinting of herpes simplex virus DNA: a novel epidemiological tool applied to a noscomial outbreak. J Infect Dis 138: 488–498

Cabrera CV, Wohlenberg C, Openshaw H, Reg-Mendez M, Puga A, Notkins AL (1980) Herpes simplex virus DNA sequences in the CNS of latently infected mice. Nature 288: 288–290

Chan WL (1983) Protective immunisation of mice with specific HSV–1 glycoproteins. Immunology 49: 343–352

Clayton AL, Roberts C, Godley M, Best JM, Chantler SM (1986) Herpes simplex virus detection by

ELISA: effect of enzyme amplification, nature of lesion sampled and specimen treatment. J Med Virol 20: 89–97

Corey L (1982) The diagnosis and treatment of genital herpes. JAMA 248: 1041–1049

Corey L (1986) Laboratory diagnosis of herpes simplex virus infections. Principles guiding the development of rapid diagnostic tests. Diagn Microbiol Infect Dis 4 (suppl 3): 111S–119S

Fife KH, Schmidt O, Remington M, Corey L (1983) Primary and recurrent concomitant genital infection with herpes simplex virus types 1 and 2. J Infect Dis 147: 163

Figuero ME, Rawls WE (1969) Biological markers for differentiation of herpes-virus strains of oral and genital origins. J Gen Virol 4: 259–267

Forghani B, Schmidt NJ, Lennette EH (1974) Solid phase radioimmunoassay for identification of herpes virus hominis type 1 and 2 from clinical materials. Appl Microbiol 28: 661–668

Frame B, Mohonty JB, Balachandron N, Rawls WE, Chernesky MA (1985) Identification and typing of herpes simplex virus by enzyme immunoassay with monoclonal antibodies. J Clin Microbiol 29: 162–166

Fraser NW, Lawrence WC, Wroblewska Z, Gilden DH, Koprowski H (1981) Herpes simplex type 1 DNA in human brain tissue. Proc Natl Acad Sci USA 78: 6461–6465

Galloway DA, Fenoglio C, Shevchuk M, McDougall JK (1979) Detection of herpes simplex RNA in human sensory ganglia. Virology 95: 265–268

Gleaves CA, Wilson DJ, Wold AD, Smith TE (1985) Detection and serotyping of herpes simplex virus in MRC-5 cells by use of centrifugation and monoclonal antibodies 16 h post inoculation. J Clin Microbiol 21: 29–32

Goldstein LC, Corey L, McDougall J, Tolentino E, Nowinski RC (1983) Monoclonal antibodies to herpes simplex viruses: use in antigenic typing and rapid diagnosis. J Infect Dis 147: 829–837

Grillner L, Landquist M (1983) Enzyme-linked immunosorbent assay for detection and typing of herpes simplex virus. Eur J Clin Microbiol 2: 39–42

Haase A, Brahic M, Stowring L. Blum H (1984) Detection of viral nucleic acids by in situ hybridisation. In: Maramorosch K, Koprowski H (Eds) Methods in virology, vol 7. Academic Press: New York, pp 189–226

Herrmann KL, Stewart JA (1981) Diagnosis of herpes simplex virus type 1 and 2 infections. In: Nahmias AJ, Dowdle WR and Schinazi RF (eds) The human herpesviruses. Elsevier, New York, pp 343–350

Hsiung GD, Landry ML, Mayo DR, Fong KY (1984a) Laboratory diagnosis of herpes simplex virus type 1 and 2 infections. Clin Dermatol 2: 67–82

Hsiung GD, Mayo DR, Landry ML, Lucia HL (1984b) Genital herpes: pathogenesis and chemotherapy in the guinea pig model. Rev Infect Dis 6: 33–50

Johnson FB, Leavitt RW, Richards DF (1985) Comparison of the Scott Selecticult-HSV kit with conventional culture and direct immunoperoxidase staining for detection of herpes simplex virus in cultures of clinical specimens. J Clin Microbiol 21: 438–441

Kelman AD, Capozza FE, Kibrick S (1975) Differential action of deoxynucleosides on mammalian cell cultures infected with herpes simplex virus types 1 and 2. J Infect Dis 131: 452–455

Lafferty WE, Krofft S, Remington M et al. (1987) Diagnosis of herpes simplex virus by direct immunofluorescence and viral isolation from samples of external genital lesions in a high prevalence population. J Clin Microbiol 25: 323–326

Land SA, Skurrie IJ, Gilbert GL (1984) Rapid diagnosis of herpes simplex virus infection by enzyme linked immunosorbent assay. J Clin Microbiol 19: 865–869

Lawrence TG, Budzko DB, Wilcke BW Jr (1984) Detection of herpes simplex virus in clinical specimens by an enzyme-linked immunosorbent assay. Am J Clin Pathol 81: 339–341

Lee FK, Coleman RM, Pereira L, Bailey PD, Tatsuno M, Nahmias AJ (1985) Detection of herpes simplex virus type 2 specific antibody with glycoprotein G. J Clin Microbiol 22: 641–644

Lee FK, Pereira L, Griffin C, Reid E, Nahmias A (1986) A novel glycoprotein for detection of herpes simplex virus type 1 specific antibodies. J Virol Methods 14:111–118

Lonsdale DM (1979) A rapid technique for distinguishing herpes-simplex virus type 1 from type 2 by restriction enzyme technology. Lancet i: 849–852

Lonsdale DM, Brown SM, Lang J, Subak-Sharpe JH, Kaprowski H, Warren KG (1980) Variations in herpes simplex virus isolated from human ganglion and a study of clonal variation in HSV 1. Ann NY Acad Sci 354: 291–308

Maniatis T, Fritsch EF, Sarnbrook J (1982) Molecular cloning: a laboratory manual. Cold Spring Harbor Laboratory Press, Cold Spring Harbour, NY.

Mayo DR, Brennan T, Egberston S H, Moore DF (1985) Rapid herpes simplex virus detection in clinical samples submitted to a state virology laboratory. J Clin Microbiol 21: 768–771

McSwiggan DA, Darougar S, Rahman AFMS, Gibson JA (1975) Comparison of the sensitivity of human embryo kidney cells, Hela cells and W1–38 cells for the primary isolation of viruses from the eye. J Clin Pathol 28: 410–413

Meinkoth J, Wahl G (1964) Hybridization of nucleic acids immobilized on solid supports. Anal Biochem 138: 267–284

Mindel A, Sutherland S (1983) Genital herpes – the disease and its treatment including intravenous acyclovir. Antimicrob Chemother 12: [suppl B]: 51–59

Minson AC, Darby G (1982) Hybridization techniques. Lab Res Methods Biol Med 5: 185–229

Morgan MA, Smith TF (1984) Evaluation of an enzyme linked immunosorbent assay for the detection of herpes simplex virus antigen. J Clin Microbiol 19: 730–732

Mosely RC. Corey L, Benjamin D, Winter C, Remington ML (1981) Comparison of viral isolation, direct immunofluorescence and indirect immunoperoxidase techniques for detection of genital herpes simplex virus infection. J Clin Microbiol 13: 913–918

Nahmias AJ, Dowdle WR (1968) Antigenic and biologic differences in herpesvirus hominis. Prog Med Virol 10: 110–159

Nahmias, AJ, Chiang WT, Del Buono I, Duffey A (1969) Typing of herpesvirus hominis strains by a direct immunofluorescent technique. Proc Soc Exp Biol Med 132: 386–390

Naib ZM (1966) Exfoliative cytology of viral cervico-vaginitis. Acta Cytol 10: 126–129

Naib ZM (1984) Cytologic diagnosis of herpes simplex virus infection. Clin Dermatol 2: 83–89

Nerurkar LS, Jacob AJ, Madden DL, Sever JL (1983) Detection of genital herpes simplex infections by a tissue culture–fluorescent-antibody technique with biotin–avidin. J Clin Microbiol 17, 149–154

Pereira L, Klassen T, Baringer J (1980) Type common and type specific monoclonal antibodies to herpes simplex virus type 1. Infect Immun 29: 724–732

Peterson E, Schmidt OW, Goldstein LC, Nowinski RC, Corey L (1983) Typing of clinical herpes simplex virus isolates with mouse monoclonal antibodies to herpes simplex virus types 1 and 2: comparison with type-specific rabbit antisera and restriction endonuclease analysis of viral DNA. J Clin Microbiol 17, 92–96

Redfield DC, Richman DD, Albanil S, Oxman MN, Wahl GM (1983) Detection of herpes simplex virus in clinical specimens by DNA hybridisation. Diagn Microbiol Infect Dis 1: 117–128

Rubin SJ, Rogers S (1984) Comparison of cultureset and primary rabbit cell cultures for the detection of herpes simplex virus. J Clin Microbiol 19: 920–922

Salmon VC, Stanberry LR, Overall JC (1984) More rapid evaluation of herpes simplex virus in a continuous line of mice lung cells than in sero or human fibroblast cells. Microbiol Infect Dis 2: 317–324

Schmidt NJ, Gallo D, Devlin V, Woodie JD, Emmons RE (1980) Direct immunofluorescence staining for detection of herpes simplex and varicella zoster virus antigens in vesicular lesions and certain tissue specimens. J Clin Microbiol 12: 651–655

Sequiera LW, Carrasco LH, Curry A, Jennings LC, Lord MA, Sutton RNP (1979) Detection of herpes simplex viral genome in brain tissue. Lancet ii: 609–612

Shekarchi IC, Sever IL, Nerurkar L, Fuccillo D (1985) Comparison of enzyme-linked immuno-sorbent assay with enzyme-linked fluorescent assay with automated readers for detection of rubella virus antibody and herpes simplex virus. Diagn Microbiol Infect Dis 21: 92–96

Sutherland S, Morgan B, Mindel A, Chan WL (1986) Typing and subtyping of herpes simplex isolates by monoclonal fluorescence. J Med Virol 18: 235–245

Unna PG (1883) On herpes progenitalis especially in women. J Cutan Genitour Dis 1: 321

Vestergaard B F, Grauballe P C (1979) ELISA for herpes simplex virus (HSV) typespecific antibodies in human sera using HSV type 1 and type 2 poly specific antigens blocked with type-heterozygous rabbit antibodies. Acta Pathol Microbiol Immunol Scand (B) 87: 261–263

Zheng ZM, Mayo DR, Hsiung ED (1983) Comparison of biological, biochemical, immunological and immunochemical techniques for typing herpes simplex virus isolates. J Clin Microbiol 17: 396–399

Chapter 8

Treatment, Prevention and Control

Introduction

The recent development of specific safe and highly efficacious chemotherapy (in particular acyclovir) has revolutionised the treatment of HSV infections. Prior to the introduction of acyclovir, treatment was limited largely to the use of extremely toxic drugs for the management of severe infections and also symptomatic treatment for the milder manifestations of the various diseases (including labial and genital herpes). In this chapter I review the pharmacology, toxicity and clinical uses of antiviral drugs for the treatment of all aspects, of HSV infection, including labial, genital, ocular, disseminated, neonatal and cerebral infections. In addition to a consideration of antiviral chemotherapy, I also review the role of immune modulation, the potential production and efficacy of vaccines to prevent genital or oral herpes, the management of genital herpes in pregnancy, the importance of health education in the control of herpes, and the management of the psychological problems associated with genital herpes.

Development of Antiherpetic drugs

In 1959 Prusoff synthesised 2′–deoxy–5–iodouridine (idoxuridine). The drug had marked antiviral activity against several DNA viruses including herpes simplex (Hermann 1961; Bauer 1977). The synthesis of idoxuridine opened the way to modern antiviral chemotherapy and, in the years that followed, several drugs were produced which had activity in vitro against HSVs.

The first generation of antiviral drugs were discovered as an offshoot of the production and subsequent testing of anticancer drugs. By and large these drugs are non-selective inhibitors of both viral and host cell replication, and as a consequence many are extremely toxic. Drugs synthesised during this phase include idoxuridine, cytosine arabinoside (cytarabine), and vidarabine.

Over recent years, scientific effort has been directed towards specific alterations in the structure of the drugs to create new preparations which inhibit the virus-specific process. Amongst the drugs produced in this way are acyclovir, bromovinyldeoxyuridine and phosphonoformic acid (Foscarnet).

Properties of the Antiviral Agents Used to Treat Herpetic Infections

Introduction

Table 8.1. lists the drugs currently used to treat herpetic infections and the clinical situations in which these drugs are used. Each of these situations will be discussed in detail below. In this section the mode of action, pharmacology and toxicity of these drugs will be reviewed.

Table 8.1. Antiviral drugs used to treat HSV infections

Drug	Uses	Comment
Acyclovir	Genital, labial, CNS, disseminated neonatal, eye	Safe and effective
Vidarabine	Neonatal, CNS, eye	Toxic systemically
Trifluorothymidine	Eye	Toxic systemically
Idoxuridine (IDU)	Eye	Toxic systemically
Bromovinyl deoxyuridine (BVDU)	Still being assessed	Still being assessed
Foscarnet (phosphonoformic acid)	Still being assessed	Still being assessed

CNS, central nervous system.

The chemical structures of the various drugs are shown in Fig. 8.1. All but one of the six drugs (Foscarnet) are nucleoside analogues.

Idoxuridine

Idoxuridine (IDU) is a synthetic halogenated pyrimidine analogue. Its antiviral activity depends on its replacement of thymidine in newly synthesised DNA (Prusoff and Ward 1976) and also on its ability, together with phosphorylated metabolites, to inhibit a variety of enzyme systems, including thymidine kinase, thymidylate synthetase, deoxycytidylate deaminase, cytidine diphosphate reductase and DNA polymerase (Muller 1979; Prusoff and Goz 1975). IDU is phosphorylated in virus-infected and uninfected host cells by deoxythymidine

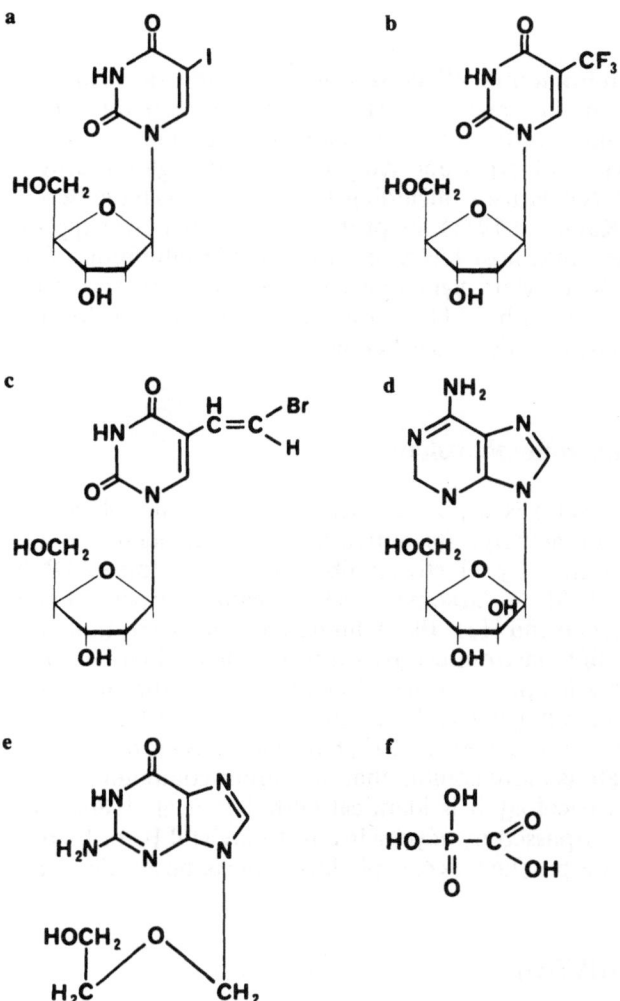

Fig. 8.1. Chemical structure of anti-herpes drugs. **a** idoxuridine. **b** trifluorothymidine. **c** Bromovinyl-deoxyuridine. **d** Vidarabine. **e** Acyclovir. **f** Phosophonoforomic acid.

kinases and successfully competes with deoxythymidine triphosphate in the DNA synthetic pathway. It is thus incorporated into the DNA of both virus-infected and normal host cells (Prusoff et al. 1979). The toxicity observed following intravenous use of this drug (mainly bone marrow depression and hepatotoxicity) is probably due to its incorporation into host DNA (Prusoff and Ward 1976). Whilst IDU is undoubtedly incorporated into host DNA, the level of incorporation into viral DNA is far higher (Prusoff and Goz 1975).

IDU established the clinical efficacy of nucleoside analogues, but its toxicity has precluded widespread use. Its only remaining use is in the treatment of eye disease (considered in detail below). However, even in this context its toxicity (oedema and photophobia) has left it as a second-line drug.

Trifluorothymidine

Trifluorothymidine (5–(trifluoromethyl)–2′–deoxyuridine) is, like idoxuridine, a synthetic halogenated pyrimidine analogue (Fig. 8.1). Its antiviral effect depends on its preferential union with viral DNA, leading to an inhibition of late viral mRNA transcription (Heidelberger and King 1979). Although the drug is active against a variety of DNA viruses, including HSV 1 and 2 (Heidelberger and King 1979; Sugar and Kaufman 1973), its profound bone marrow suppression, due to its incorporation into host DNA and irreversible inhibition of an essential DNA percusor, thymidylate synthetase (Prusoff and Ward 1976), precludes its systemic use. As with IDU its only remaining use is for the management of ocular herpetic infections (see below).

Vidarabine and Vidarabine Monophosphate

Vidarabine (adenine arabinoside) is a purine nucleoside analogue which has both antiviral and anticancer activity. Its antiviral activity depends on the suppression of viral DNA synthesis by selective inhibition of virus-induced DNA polymerases (Muller 1977, 1979). Vidarabine is active against herpes simplex but its poor solubility (Buchanan and Hess 1980), limited topical absorption, and considerable toxicity (including gastrointestinal disorders, hallucinations, tremor, dysarthria, bone marrow suppression, hepatotoxity, rashes, thrombophlebitis and possible teratogenic, mutagenic and carcinogenic effects: Whitley et al. 1976, 1982; Van Etta et al. 1981; Bodey et al. 1975) has limited its usefulness.

   Vidarabine monophosphate is more soluble than its parent compound but in all other aspects including toxicology it is identical (Whitley et al. 1980a). Its usefulness has largely been surpassed by acyclovir but it may still be of help in some patients with neonatal herpes, herpes encephalitis or herpetic eye disease.

Bromovinyldeoxyuridine (BVDU)

BVDU is another purine analogue with a very marked and highly specific effect against herpes simplex viruses, HSV 1 in particular (De Clercq et al. 1979). Its antiviral effect depends on its phosphorylation, in cells infected by HSV, by an HSV-induced thymidine kinase (TK) (Cheng et al. 1981). The drug appears to have a high affinity for TK induced by HSV 1 but not that induced by HSV 2 (Cheng et al. 1981). The difference in antiviral effect between HSV 1 and 2 appears to be due to selective phosphorylation of BVDU–5′–monophosphate by the HSV 1–induced TK (Fyfe 1982). The drug is apparently well absorbed orally (De Clercq 1985). As yet, little is known of its clinical efficacy and toxicity.

Acyclovir

Acyclovir (2–amino–1,9–dihydro–9[2–hydroxyethoxy)methyl]–6H–purin–6–one) is a purine analogue of deoxyguanine. As with the other such analogues, its activity depends on suppression of viral DNA synthesis. Its mechanism of action

Fig. 8.2. Mechanisms of action of acyclovir. The drug acts at three points. (1) Competition with deoxyguanine for thymidine kinase. (2) Competition for DNA polymerase. (3) DNA chain termination.

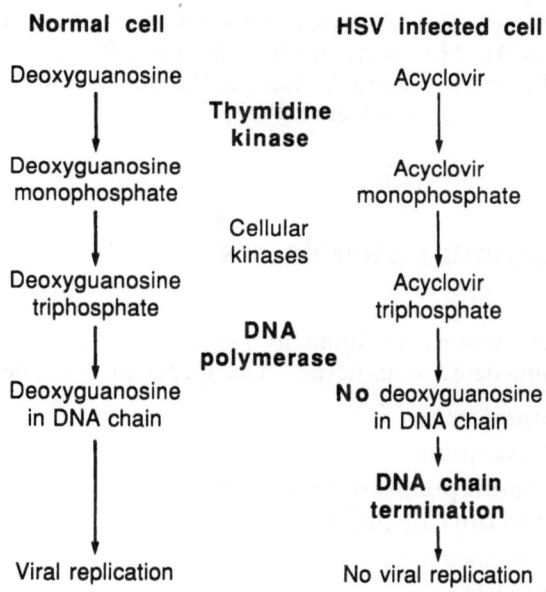

has been studied in depth and it is known that the drug or its phosphorylated derivatives act on several points in the DNA synthetic pathway (Fig. 8.2).

Acyclovir competes as a substrate with the deoxynucleosides and is selectively phosphorylated by viral thymidine kinase (Elion 1982). Viral TK is far more effective than cellular TK in phosphorylating acyclovir. Therefore the active drug targets infected as opposed to uninfected cells. Acyclovir monophosphate is converted to its di- and triphosphate derivatives by cellular enzymes (Miller and Miller 1980). Acyclovir triphosphate is the active metabolite of the drug. It acts by competing selectively with the deoynucleoside triphosphates for viral DNA polymerase (Furman et al. 1979) and more importantly by its inhibitory effect on DNA polymerase (Elion 1982),. The substrate activity of acyclovir triphosphate is self-limiting, as the incorporated acyclovir monophosphate lacks a 3'–OH group, which results in DNA chain termination (Furman et al. 1979).

Acyclovir is highly effective against HSVs. Clinical trials suggest that the drug is efficient in the treatment of oral, genital, ocular and disseminated infections. These will be considered in detail below. The drug, although poorly absorbed, is effective orally. Toxicity is minimal. Transient renal dysfunction may occur in dehydrated individuals, or in those with pre-existing renal disease, or where the drug is given as an intravenous bolus injection (Mindel et al. 1982; Weller et al. 1983). Other side-effects appear to be rare and of little clinical importance.

Phosphonoformic Acid (Foscarnet)

Unlike all the above-mentioned drugs, Foscarnet is not a nucleoside analogue (Fig. 8.1). Its mode of action depends on selective inhibition of viral DNA polymerase (Huang et al. 1976; Mao and Robishaw 1975). There have been only a few clinical studies to assess its efficacy. Topical therapy for labial and genital herpes does not look too promising (Sacks et al. 1987; Wallin et al. 1985; Öberg 1983). However, further studies will be needed to confirm these results. Parenteral therapy may be limited by toxicity, damage to the kidneys in particular (Gaub et al. 1987).

Immune Modulators

A number of immune modulators have been used to treat patients with mucocutaneous herpes. The agents are listed below:

Interferons
Levamisole
Inosine pranobex (isoprinosine)
TP5 (thymopentin)
Vaccines
    BCG
    Smallpox
    Polio
    Influenza
    Yellow Fever

The use of these drugs has been extensively reviewed elsewhere (Overall 1984; Mindel and Sutherland 1983; Corey 1985; Corey and Spear 1986), and the overall picture that emerges is that none of the agents has any significant effect on mucocutaneous herpes.

One drug, inosine pranobex (Isoprinosine) warrants some further discussion. Several reports suggested that this might be useful in the treatment of genital or oral herpes (Corey et al. 1979; W. H. Wickett, L. J. Bradshaw, J. Wilson and A. J. Galasky, 1976, unpublished results; Galli et al. 1982; Salo and Lassus 1983; Bouffat and Saurat 1980). A recent study conducted in our unit, with co-workers from the Royal Hallamshire Hospital in Sheffield, in patients with first-attack genital herpes, suggests that this is not the case (Mindel et al. 1987). Seventy-seven patients with a first attack of genital herpes were treated with acyclovir or inosine pranobex, or both, in a randomised placebo-controlled study. Those treated with acyclovir (either on its own or in combination) healed more quickly and had a shorter duration of symptoms and viral excretion than those treated with inosine pranobex alone. We have recently completed a study comparing the efficacy of inosine pranobex with acyclovir for the suppression of frequently recurring genital herpes. The study showed that acyclovir is vastly superior to inosine pranobex (Mindel et al. 1989).

Finally, a recent study has suggested that topical interferon may reduce the frequency and severity of outbreaks in patients with oral or genital herpes (Glezerman et al. 1988). Further trials will be required to confirm these findings.

Table 8.2. Miscellaneous therapies suggested for the treatment of HSV infections

Topical surfactants	Topical steroids
Ether	Methyl alcohol
Chloroform	Gentian violet
Nonoxynol 9	Copper sulphate
Thymol	Potassium permanganate
Photodynamic inactivation	Boric acid ointment
Neutral red	Urea
Proflavine	Tannic acid ointment
Lysine	Vitamin E, C and B12
2'-Deoxy-D-glucose	Ginseng
Zinc	Aloe vera extracts
Lithium	Red algae
Dimethyl sulphoxide (DMSO)	Laser therapy
Povidine jodine	Cryotherapy
Oral and/or topical antibiotics	

Non-specific Therapies

There are numerous non-specific therapies that have been tried for the treatment of mucocutaneous herpes (Table 8.2). As with the immune modulators, these have been extensively reviewed (Overall 1984; Corey 1985, 1986; Adler and Mindel 1985; Mindel and Sutherland 1983) and again the overall picture that emerges is that none of these agents has any effect. More recent work with several agents warrants some discussion. Two triterpenoid compounds, carbenoxolone and cicloxclone, have been studied for the treatment of mucocutaneous herpes. Both drugs are derivatives of glycyrrhetic acid, a substance derived from the root of the liquorice plant (Dargan and Subak-Sharpe 1986). Carbenoxolone is used for the management of gastric and duodenal ulceration. Carbenoxolone has been reported from open studies to benefit patients with orolabial herpes (Poswillo and Roberts 1981; Partridge and Poswillo 1984). However, only one placebo-controlled trial has been reported. This was a study in patients with genital herpes (Csonka and Tyrrell 1984). Although the study suggested that patients treated with both preparations healed more quickly, with a shorter duration of pain than in placebo recipients, this study has a number of flaws that make interpretation of the results difficult. Firstly, the authors combined patients with first-attack disease and those with recurrences. As the clinical features of these two aspects of genital herpes are so different (see Chap. 4) this is clearly inappropriate. Other problems with the study include a large number of exclusions , and no virological data.

A topical surfactant 'Inter-VirA' (a combination of p-diisobutylphenoxy-polyethoxyethanol and polyoxyethylene–10–oleyl ether) has recently been reported to be efficacious in patients with recurrent genital herpes (Goldberg 1986). The results of this study have been criticised for poor statistical analysis and lack of objective measures (Gold et al. 1986). An additional problem is that the authors failed to use the best measure of efficacy, namely the effect on the duration of viral excretion. It is also of interest that studies with other topical surfactants in both oral and genital herpes have not shown any significant clinical benefit (Corey et al. 1978; Vontver et al. 1979; Farrell and Nesland 1977; Taylor et al. 1977).

Treatment of Ocular Herpes

The major objective in treating herpetic eye disease is to preserve vision. Each of the different anatomical areas of the eye infected with HSV requires a different strategy of treatment and each will be considered in turn.

Blepharitis and Conjunctivitis

Herpetic infection of the periorbital skin, eyelids and conjunctiva is usually seen as part of the primary illness, although recurrence at this site can occur from time to time. Where the cornea is not involved, the use of topical antiviral therapy is recommended (McGill and Scott 1985; Dawson 1984; Pavan-Langston 1984). However, there are no trials comparing antivirals in this situation and acyclovir, trifluorothymidine, vidarabine and IDU are probably all suitable, although the toxicity of the last two agents limits their usefulness.

Keratitis

The three types of keratitis (infectious ulcers, trophic or non-infectious ulcers and finally stromal disease (see Chap. 4) each require a different therapeutic approach.

Infectious ulcers are the simplest to treat. Debridment alone shortens the course of the illness (Jones et al. 1976), and the subsequent application of topical antivirals eliminates virus from the cornea (Dawson 1984). Several antivirals (acyclovir, trifluorothymidine, vidarabine and IDU) are effective; and clinical trials (Coster et al. 1979, 1983; McCulley et al. 1982; Collum et al. 1980; Colin et al. 1981; McGill et al 1981; Young et al. 1982; La Lau et al. 1982) do not give a clear picture of a single drug with superior efficacy. Less toxicity with acyclovir and trifluorothymidine probably favour their use.

The epithelial (non-infectious or metaherpetic) ulcers are considerably more difficult to manage. Daily applications of antivirals and antibiotics to prevent secondary infection, followed by a firm dressing or the use of a soft contact lense, is recommended (Pavan-Langston 1984; Dawson 1984).

Stromal keratitis is the most difficult form of keratitis to manage. Topical steroids have long been used in this condition to suppress the inflammatory response. The problems with steroids include the enhancement or production of infectious epithelial ulcers (Patterson and Jones 1967), a rebound in stromal infiltration after stopping therapy, and the development of bacterial or fungal superinfection, glaucoma or even cataracts (McGill and Scott 1985). Consequently topical antivirals are always used in conjunction with steroids. The only antiviral to penetrate the eye is acyclovir. In patients with no previous exposure to steroids, topical acyclovir appears to be highly successful (McGill 1984), but in those where steroids have been used, success with acyclovir alone is limited. The combination of acyclovir with topical steroids seems to have a high cure rate (Collum et al. 1983). There is some interest in the use of systemic acyclovir (with or without topical preparations) to treat the condition.

Iridocyclitis

The traditional treatment of deep-seated herpetic eye disease involves the use of cytoplegic mydriatics and topical antivirals (Pavan-Langston 1984; Dawson 1984). Acyclovir, with its ability to penetrate the eye, is the antiviral of choice and again, as with stromal disease, there is interest in the use of systemic acyclovir (L. M. T. Collum, unpublished work presented at Wellcome Internat Antiviral Symp, Monte Carlo, 2–4 December 1987). Steroids should be avoided if possible, but as with stromal keratitis, once steroids have been commenced, patients may become steroid dependent.

In all forms of herpetic eye disease the use of antivirals does not prevent recurrences. Whether suppressive antiviral therapy (as used in immunosuppressed patients or patients with frequently recurring genital herpes, see below) would prevent recurrences has not yet been established. This is an exciting possibility in patients with frequent recurrences.

Choroidoretinitis

Herpes simplex choroidoretinitis occurs in immunocompromised patients and infants with neonatal herpes (see Chap. 5). The treatment of disseminated, and neonatal HSV is discussed below.

Treatment of Orolabial Herpes

In order to assess the efficacy of any therapy one requires measurable parameters. Many of these may be highly subjective (e.g. the assessment of symptoms), whereas others are more objective (e.g. healing times or the duration of virus excretion) and consequently easier to measure and to compare. Prior to conducting or assessing the results of clinical trials, the aims of treatment should be clearly delineated. In both primary and recurrent orolabial herpes the aims of treatment are to hasten healing, shorten the duration of symptoms (including pain, itching and fever) and, to reduce the duration of virus excretion (Overall 1984). Perhaps the most important objective and the one most difficult to achieve is to prevent the development of latency. Finally, it is vital to use randomised double-blind placebo-controlled studies to assess the efficacy of any new treatment (Brigden 1985; Overall 1984).

Primary Orolabial Herpes

Despite the fact that primary orolabial herpes is a relatively common and severe illness, there are no controlled trials of antivirals in this condition. Such studies are awaited with interest. Until these results are available, the most suitable antiviral would seem to be acyclovir. As the illness is often systemic, a 5-day course of oral acyclovir is probably advisable.

In patients with severe gingivostomatitis, symptomatic therapy is most important. Patients should be given adequate analgesia and attention should be given
to the maintenance of good oral hygiene. Many young children will refuse to eat
and care should be taken to ensure that an adequate fluid intake is given.

Recurrent Orolabial Herpes

In contrast to the situation in primary orolabial herpes, in the recurrent condition
a plethora of therapies have been tested. These preparations have been reviewed
(Overall 1984; Pazin and Harger 1986). Of the 19 preparations listed by Overall
(1984), five were not tested in double-blind placebo-controlled trials (smallpox
and influenza vaccines, povidone-iodine, zinc sulphate and cryotherapy). The
results with the other 14 preparations (IDU, cytosine arabinoside, adenine
arabinoside, acyclovir, phosphonoformic acid, kethoxal cream, photodynamic
inactivation, ether, chloroform, lysine, levamisole, interferons, bioflavonoids and
ascorbic acid, and boric acid) were by and large disappointing. The use of
acyclovir does warrant some further consideration. Two different formulations of
topical acyclovir have been evaluated in double-blind placebo-controlled studies –
acyclovir ointment in a polyethylene glycol base (Spruance et al. 1982; Raborn et
al. 1988) and acyclovir cream in a propylene glycol base (Fiddian et al. 1983a;
Fiddian and Ivanyi 1983; Shaw et al. 1985; Raborn et al. 1988). Two of the studies
(Fiddian and Ivanyi 1983; Fiddian et al. 1983a), both using acyclovir cream,
suggested that healing times were shorter in patients treated with acyclovir, but
the remainder of the studies have not confirmed this. The original suggestion that
these differences could be explained on the basis of the different formulations, no
longer appears tenable, as lack of efficacy has now been demonstrated in trials
with both.

What about oral acyclovir? The only placebo-controlled trial reported to date
suggested that patients treated with acyclovir healed more quickly and had a
shorter duration of viral excretion and symptoms than those who received
placebo (Raborn et al. 1988). It is worth noting that these effects, although
statistically significant, were only of marginal clinical benefit. At present,
treating episodes of labial herpes with short courses of topical or oral acyclovir
does not appear to be warranted.

A novel approach to the problem is the use of acyclovir to suppress or prevent
recurrences. A double-blind trial treating patients with 16 weeks of twice-daily
topical acyclovir or placebo showed no differences between the two preparations
(Fawcett et al. 1983). In contrast, suppressive oral acyclovir does appear to
prevent recurrences. During 12 weeks of a double-blind placebo-controlled trial
in patients with recurrent labial herpes, only 2 out of 12 acyclovir recipients
compared with 9 out of 12 placebo recipients suffered a recurrence (P=0.0016)
(Meyrick Thomas et al. 1985). Spruance (1988) has recently reported on the
efficacy of prophylactic acyclovir to prevent recurrences in patients exposed to
ultraviolet light, both as a natural occurrence (e.g. whilst skiing) and also in the
laboratory. In both these circumstances, acyclovir can prevent or reduce the
frequency of recurrences. Acyclovir has been reported also to prevent recurrences occurring as a result of trigeminal surgery (Schädelin et al. 1988).

In summary, suppressive oral acyclovir may be a useful treatment for patients
with frequent recurrences of oro-labial herpes or may be used to prevent

recurrences during periods where patients are likely to develop them (e.g. exposure to ultraviolet light or surgery).

Treatment of Genital Herpes

The clinical features of genital herpes are very similar to those of orolabial herpes, but there are several aspects of the illness which make management more complicated, including the associated psychosexual morbidity and the fact that many individuals have frequent recurrences (see Chap. 4). As with orolabial herpes, the parameters for "measuring success" in both first-attack and recurrent herpes include the assessment of symptoms, the time to healing, duration of virus excretion and the prevention of recurrences. Treatment of the first attack and the treatment and suppression of recurrences will be considered separately.

First-Attack Genital Herpes

Numerous treatments have been suggested for first-attack genital herpes and these have been reviewed extensively (Belsey and Adler 1978; Mindel and Sutherland 1983; Mindel 1984; Adler and Mindel 1985; Overall 1984; Corey 1986).

Acyclovir is the only drug out of the plethora of suggested therapies that has been shown in a series of randomised, double-blind placebo-controlled studies to have any consistent clinical and virological benefit in this condition. Intravenous, oral and topical acyclovir have all been tested (Mindel et al. 1982; Corey et al. 1982, 1983; Nilsen et al. 1982; Bryson et al. 1983; Mertz et al. 1984; Kinghorn et al. 1983; Thin et al. 1983; Fiddian et al. 1983b). All three preparations have some clinical effect, although parenteral therapy seems to be more effective than topical. This is not surprising as first-attack genital herpes is a systemic illness (see Chap. 4). Other theoretical advantages of systemic therapy include prevention (or treatment) of meningitis, optimum therapeutic drug levels delivered to all anatomical sites, and the ability to reach all infected sites (including the cervix, anal canal and urethra).

The majority of patients can be adequately managed as out-patients with oral therapy. Treatment with oral acyclovir (200 mg, five times daily) for 10 days (Bryson et al. 1983; Mertz et al. 1984) does not appear to be any better than 5 days of treatment (Nilsen et al. 1982).

One of the disappointing aspects of treatment has been the observation that acyclovir does not prevent the development of recurrences or decrease their frequency (Mertz et al. 1984; Corey et al. 1985). Even prolonged treatment of the first attack does not achieve this objective (Mindel et al. 1986). This is not surprising, as animal experiments suggest that latency is established within 48 h of exposure (see Chap. 2) and treatment is often not commenced until considerably later. As acyclovir is only effective against replicating virus, latent virions remain unaffected.

In addition to antiviral chemotherapy patients also require symptomatic treatment and psychosexual support. Mild analgesia (e.g. aspirin or paraceta-mol) are usually adequate to control the pain and fever. Frequent bathing in dilute saline keeps the area clean and is often very soothing. Application of ice packs may also be helpful. Women with severe dysuria may find that urination is easier in the bath. Occasionally patients with urinary retention require catheri-sation, although in our experience early treatment with acyclovir often prevents this.

As mentioned in Chap. 4, many patients have psychosexual problems associated with herpes. Sympathetic management, knowledgeable advice and prolonged support are often required (Derman 1986). One of the most difficult problems to deal with is when genital herpes occurs in one of the partners of the stable relationship. Reassurances about fidelity and detailed information about the mode of transmission are vital.

Treatment and Suppression of Recurrences

As with first attack herpes, the assortment of treatments that have been tested or suggested for the treatment of recurrences is vast, and again, as with first-attack genital herpes the only drug that has been shown to have an effect is acyclovir (Nilsen et al. 1982; Salo et al. 1983; Corey et al. 1982; Fiddian et al. 1983b; Kinghorn et al. 1983; Reichman et al. 1984). Although these studies showed that there was a statistically significant reduction in the duration of virus excretion and the time to healing, the actual relevance of this to patient management is questionable. Most of the studies showed that healing times were approximately one day shorter in the acyclovir recipients compared with controls, and taking tablets or using cream for 5 days to reduce the duration of the illness from 6 days to 5 is at best a marginal benefit. Using the treatment as early as possible in the attack does appear to be somewhat better (Reichman et al. 1984) and may be suitable management for patients with infrequent attacks.

Another approach is to use continuous suppressive acyclovir to prevent recurrences. Several studies have shown that this is a highly effective form of therapy (Fig. 8.3; see also Douglas et al. 1984; Straus et al. 1984; Mindel et al. 1984; Thin et al. 1985; Halsos et al. 1985; Kinghorn et al. 1985) and continuous use of the drug can suppress recurrences for prolonged periods. Studies we have recently completed suggest that the drug is safe and that patients should be commenced on therapy of 200 mg four times a day. If after 2–3 months the patient is recurrence free, the dosage can be reduced to 200 mg thrice daily and then to 200 mg twice daily. Some patients may even be controlled on one 200 mg tablet daily (Fig. 8.4; see also Mindel et al. 1988). Several important questions remain to be answered about this form of treatment, the most vexing one being "who should be treated?" Patients with one or more recurrences per month would certainly be suitable whereas those with one or two a year would not. Where one draws the line between these two extremes is a matter of clinical judgement and discussion between doctor and patient. Other factors important in reaching a decision include the duration and severity of recurrences, the likelihood of spread to a sexual partner, and any associated psychological or psychosexual morbidity. The second important question is "how long should treatment continue?" Acyclovir is certainly effective for at least 2 years (Mertz

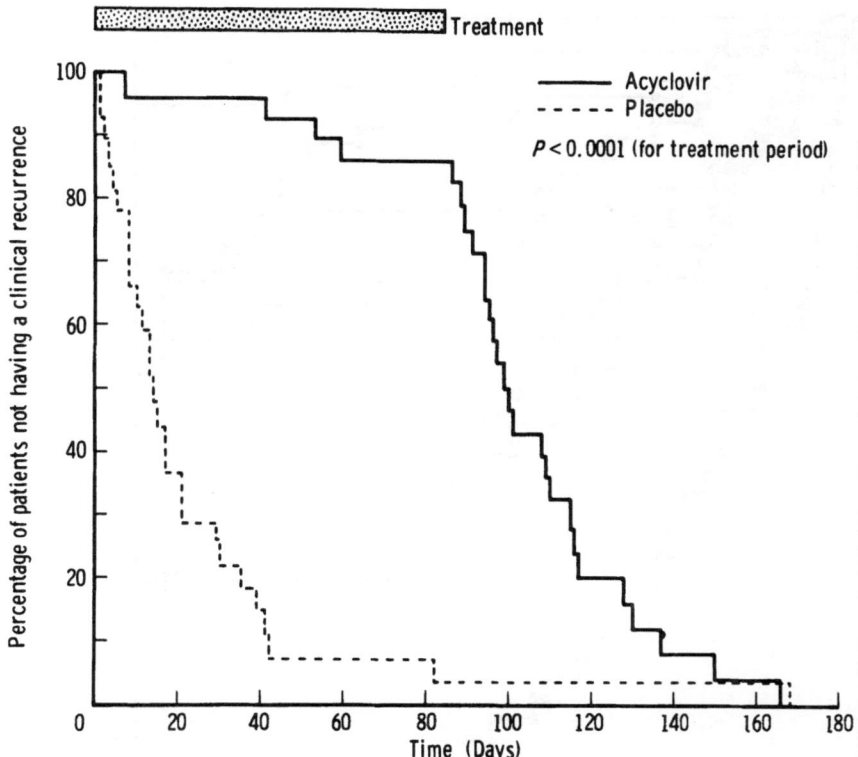

Fig. 8.3. Suppression of recurrent genital herpes. Time to first recurrence, comparing patients treated for 12 weeks in a randomised double-blind study with acyclovir or placebo. Of the acyclovir recipients, 14% recurred during treatment, compared with 98% of the placebo recipients: $P<0.0001$. (From Mindel et al. 1984.)

et al. 1988); however, recent evidence suggested that after one year of therapy the frequency of recurrences may be significantly reduced (Mindel et al. 1988). It would seem prudent therefore to stop treatment after one year and reassess the situation.

Prevention and Treatment of Neonatal Herpes

Prevention

The majority of cases of neonatal herpes are acquired at the time of delivery from the infected birth canal. In 1971 Nahmias et al. in Atlanta, Georgia, reported that neonatal herpes could be prevented if the baby was delivered by Caesarian section (CS) rather than through the infected birth canal. Although CS is now widely recommended if the mother has herpes at term, this form of

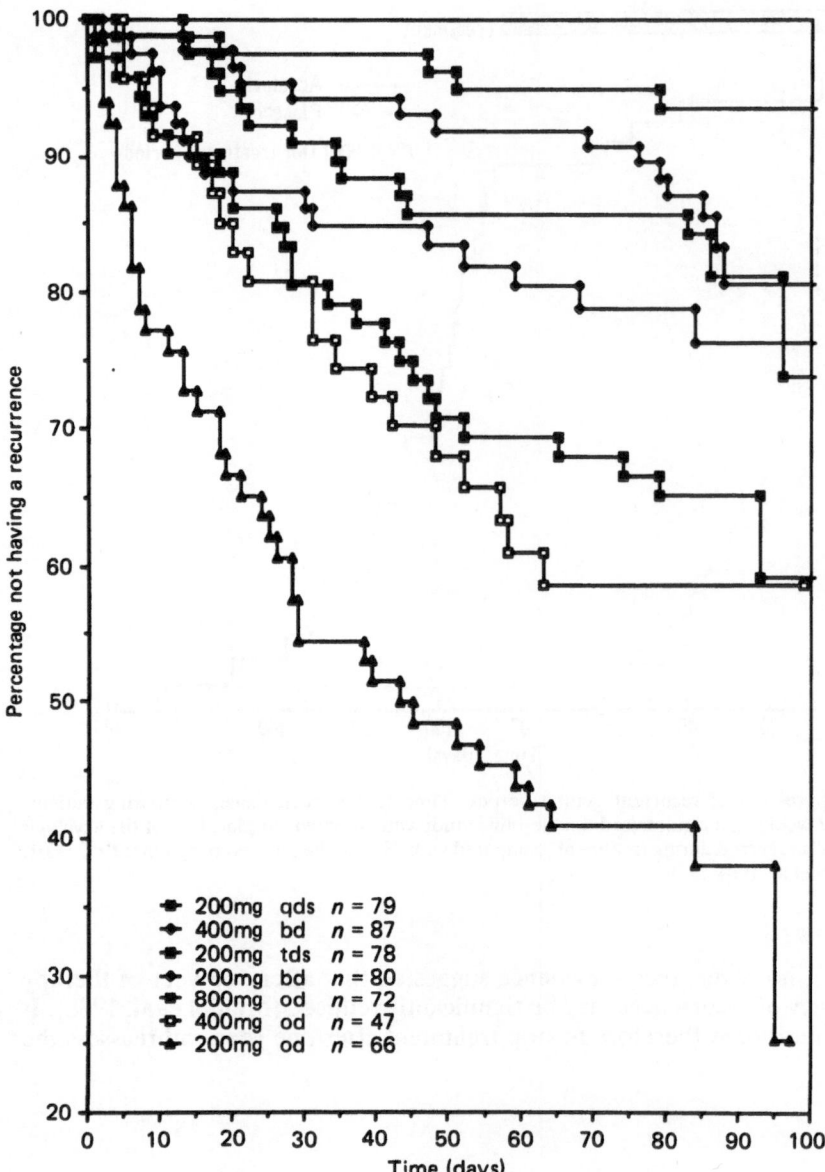

Fig. 8.4. The time to first recurrence in patients with frequently recurring genital herpes, comparing various dosages of acyclovir.
The more frequent the dosage the less likely the patient is to recur.
qds, four times daily; bd, twice daily; tds, thrice daily; od, once daily. (From Mindel et al. 1988).

therapy remains unproven in controlled clinical trials. If the mother has primary herpes at term, the risk that the neonate (with no protective maternal antibodies and high viral titres) will develop herpes is certainly high (Brown et al. 1987; Nahmias and Keyserling 1984). In this circumstance CS is to be recommended.

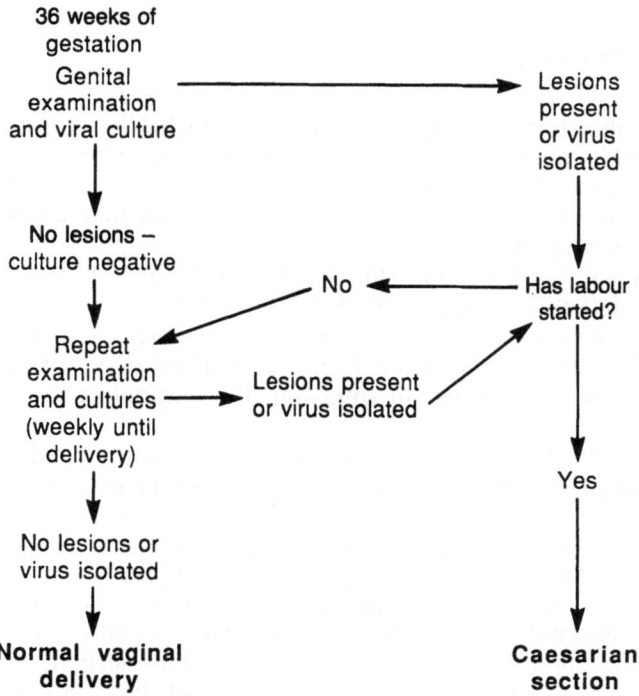

Fig. 8.5. Screening for herpes in pregnancy.

The situation in regard to recurrent herpes is entirely different. Firstly, the risks of the neonate developing herpes following delivery through an infected birth canal in a mother with recurrent herpes is estimated to be less than 5% (Binkin et al. 1984; Prober et al. 1987) and, secondly, CS itself has an associated mortality and morbidity (Binkin et al. 1984).

In order to perform CS, women with HSV infection at term need to be identified. The method used is to examine the genitalia and take viral cultures every week from all women with a history of genital herpes (or with a current sexual partner who has herpes), from 34 or 36 weeks of pregnancy till delivery (Commitee on Fetus and Newborn 1980). CS is recommended if at the onset of labour the most recent viral culture was positive or if lesions suggestive of herpes are present (Fig. 8.5). This form of screening has a number of disadvantages:

Advantages
1. Confirms suspected lesions
2. Detects some cases of inapparent HSV lesions or viral shedding
3. Reassures patient
4. Reassures doctor

Disadvantages
1. May not be necessary
2. Will miss cases without a history of previous herpes

3. Expense
4. Caesarian section has a morbidity and mortality.

It will not detect women who shed virus asymptomatically but who have never had clinical herpes, nor will it detect patients who shed virus between visits. It is extremely costly (Binkin et al. 1984), time consuming and requires the patient to make several additional visits to the doctor. Also, viral cultures may take up to one week to show the changes typical of HSV.

Several studies have shown that a considerable number of mothers transmit HSV to their infants without being aware that they themselves have herpes (Whitley et al. 1980b; Sullivan-Bolyai et al. 1983). The newly described type-specific assays to detect HSV 2 and HSV 1 antibodies (Lee et al. 1985, 1986) may be a useful screening test to use in antenatal clinics to detect these inapparent infections.

Is there any alternative to CS? At the present time the answer is no, but the possible use of antiviral drugs (in particular acyclovir) in later pregnancy in 'at risk' mothers is being considered (Mindel 1984). Over and above the obvious problem of deciding who should be treated, two further problems remain. Is the drug safe in late pregnancy and is it efficacious? Limited safety data from women who have taken the drug inadvertently in pregnancy look encouraging (Andrews et al. 1988), but more detailed studies are required. The question of efficacy will be resolved only with carefully controlled trials. The conduct of such trials involves a number of difficult ethical issues, including the use of drugs in late pregnancy (allbeit the third trimester) and whether CS should still be performed.

Treatment

In the absence of treatment, neonatal herpes has a 60% mortality and many of the surviving infants are profoundly disabled (see Chap. 5). Vidarabine and acyclovir are both useful drugs for the treatment of neonatal herpes, randomised, double-blind placebo-controlled trials have shown that vidarabine reduces mortality from 74% to 38%. However, a considerable number of infants who survive are left with residual neurological problems, including microcephaly, hemiparesis, seizures, spasticity and blindness (Whitley et al. 1980b).

A recently reported study comparing the efficacy of vidarabine with acyclovir (Whitley 1988) showed that the efficacy of the two preparations was similar. Both drugs reduced mortality, but in the survivors residual problems were common, especially in the babies with central nervous system or disseminated infections. Corey et al. (1988) have shown that the neurological outcome of herpetic encephalitis in neonates is dependent on viral type. Patients with HSV 2 are more likely to have long-term problems (including microcephaly, seizures, cerebral palsy, mental retardation and eye defects) irrespective of whether they received acyclovir or vidarabine.

The response to therapy in neonates is disappointing. Antivirals decrease mortality, but some neurological problems often remain. The reasons for the relatively poor response are unclear. Improved strategies for detection, prevention and treatment are required.

Encephalitis

Both vidarabine and acyclovir are useful drugs for the treatment of HSV encephalitis. Vidarabine, first evaluated in the 1970s, appeared to reduce mortality at 6 months from 70% to 30% (Whitley et al. 1977). Further studies showed that mortality or morbidity was related to several other factors, irrespective of treatment (Whitley et al. 1982). Older patients, those who were semiconscious or comatose and those with longer periods prior to the onset of therapy had a worse prognosis than the younger patients, those with higher levels of consciousness and those in whom therapy was started earlier. Taking the two extremes 6 months after presentation, almost 80% of comatose patients over 30 years of age treated with vidarabine, will be dead, whereas fewer than 10% of patients under 30 years, treated with vidarabine, who were lethargic will have died.

Two trials have compared the efficacy of acyclovir with vidarabine. Both were well-conducted, randomised and controlled but not double-blind (Sweden – Sköldenberg et al. 1984; USA – Whitley et al. 1986). The results from both trials were broadly comparable. Overall mortality in the acyclovir group at 6 months was 19% in the Swedish study and 28% in the American study and in vidarabine recipients it varied from 50% to 54%. Older patients and those with a higher coma score were more likely to die and those that survived often had moderate or severe neurological impairment.

It is evident from these studies that acyclovir is the drug of choice. The recommended dos is 10 mg kg^{-1}, 8 hourly by slow intravenous infusion for 10 days. Every effort should be made to treat as early as possible.

The debate regarding brain biopsy remains unresolved (see Chap. 5). However, if herpes is considered to be a possible diagnosis it would seem prudent to commence patients on acyclovir immediately. Any subsequent biopsy will still be able to diagnose other conditions which may be considered in the differential diagnosis. The only drawback with this recommendation is that some cases of herpes will not be confirmed, as acyclovir may interfere with virus culture.

Treatment of Severe Mucocutaneous and Disseminated Herpes

Severe herpetic infections in immunocompromised patients may threaten the life of the individual. Antiviral chemotherapy, with acyclovir in particular, has revolutionised treatment in this context.

Several trials have shown that acyclovir is a highly effective treatment for immunocompromised patients with severe mucocutaneous and disseminated herpes simplex infections (Mitchell et al. 1981; Chou et al. 1981; Wade et al. 1982; Meyers et al. 1982). Most of these studies used intravenous acyclovir; in life-threatening or severe infections, or in patients where oral absorption might be a problem, this approach is entirely appropriate. The recommended dose is

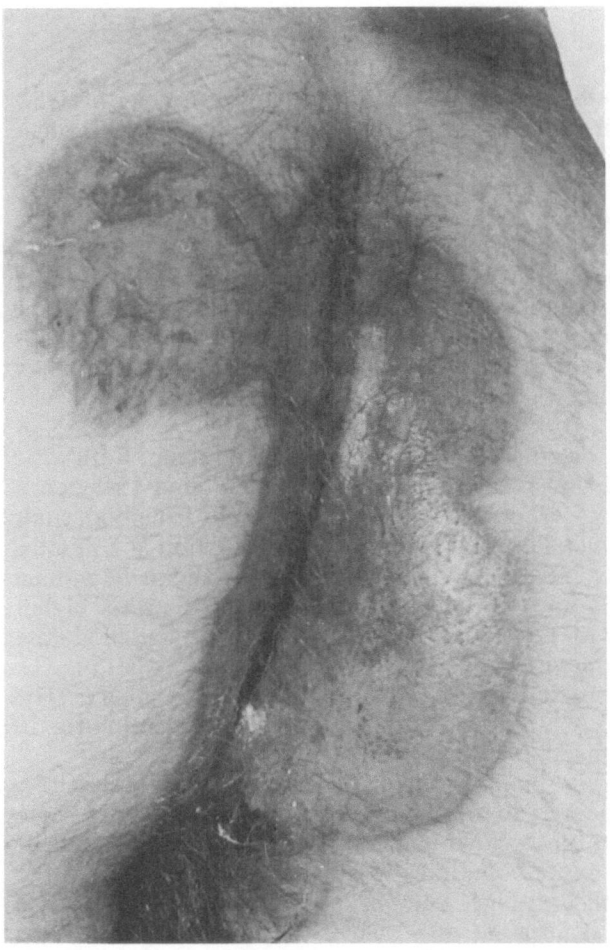

Fig. 8.6. Healing of extensive perianal ulceration in an AIDS patient following 10 days of intravenous acyclovir. (See Fig. 5.5. (p. 84) for the clinical appearance before treatment.)

10 mg kg^{-1}, 8 hourly, by slow infusion. In patients with less severe infections oral therapy may be acceptable.

Although controlled trials have not been conducted in patients with the acquired immunodeficiency syndrome (AIDS), our own experience and other anecdotal reports suggest that acyclovir is equally effective in this situation (Fig. 8.6).

Another approach is the use of acyclovir as a prophylactic to prevent viral reactivation and the development of clinical lesions. This has proved highly effective in bone marrow transplant recipients and cancer patients receiving chemotherapy (Saral et al. 1981, 1983; Hann et al. 1983; Wade et al. 1984). In many of these patients herpes can be successfully suppressed with oral acyclovir, 400 mg, five times daily. Whether suppression can still be achieved with lower doses remains to be determined. Our own uncontrolled experience in patients infected with the human immunodeficiency virus (HIV) suggests that 200 mg, four times daily, may be equally successful.

The relationship between HSV and dermatological conditions is discussed in Chap. 5. Although fewer studies have been conducted in patients with these complaints, the small number that have been done, as well as anecdotal reports, suggest that acyclovir may again have an important part to play. In patients (usually children) with eczema herpeticum, acyclovir (oral if less severe, intravenous in more severe cases) may be life-saving. Patients with recurrences can usually be managed with oral acyclovir. Suppression of frequently recurring eczema herpeticum may again be achieved with oral acyclovir.

Several recent reports have shown that oral acyclovir can be used with considerable success to prevent herpes attacks in patients with erythema multiforme (Fawcett et al. 1983; Leigh 1988). These studies are particularly interesting in that they show that acyclovir prevents erythema multiforme not only in those with preceding episodes of orolabial herpes, but also in those without and suggest that subclinical herpes may be the precipitating factor in many patients with no obvious trigger for their erythema multiforme. In such patients a therapeutic trial with suppressive oral acyclovir may be useful.

Failure to Respond to Acyclovir Treatment

The majority of patients treated with acyclovir respond to therapy, but a small number fail to do so. There are several reasons for failure of therapy including patients not taking the drug or taking an insufficient dose, malabsorption (Mindel and Carney 1988), the condition due to some other pathology, and finally resistance to therapy.

Resistance can result from alteration in two loci on the HSV genome – the regions coding for thymidine kinase (TK) and DNA polymerase enzymes (Coen and Schaffer 1981; Schnipper and Crumpacker 1980; Field et al. 1980). Viruses with reduced sensitivity to acyclovir (mostly TK-negative strains) have been reported, although the number of reports is small and mostly in immunocompromised patients who have received long or repeated courses of therapy (Burns et al. 1982; Crumpacker et al. 1982; Sibrack et al. 1982; Wade et al. 1983; Schinazi et al. 1986). A handful of reports suggests that resistant isolates may rarely be found in patients with normal immunity – even prior to the administration of acyclovir (McClaren et al. 1983; Straus et al. 1984). It is of interest that recovery of resistant virus may not correlate with a poor clinical response, and that virus isolated from patients with previously demonstrated resistant strains may be sensitive to subsequent treatment.

Although resistance remains uncommon, vigilance will be required to see that it remains so. It is interesting to postulate "biological situations" that may be likely to give rise to resistant strains. Repeated courses of treatment using suboptimal doses (e.g. repeated courses of topical acyclovir for recurrent oral or genital herpes) may favour the emergence of such strains; whereas suppressive therapy (in sufficient dose) may prevent their emergence by stopping viral replication. TK-negative strains occur spontaneously and are probably eliminated by the immune system; however, in immunosuppressed patients this may not occur. Making sure that immunosuppressed patients receive adequate acyclovir doses to prevent reactivation may be important.

Prevention of Herpetic Infections

Introduction

There are several approaches to the prevention of herpes and these are listed below:

1. Education
   Increase in public awareness about HSV
   Increase in professional awareness about HSV
2. Decrease exposure
   Use of condoms
   Awareness about infectivity
   Pregnancy screening
3. Antiviral prophylaxis
4. Vaccines

Health education to encourage public awareness about the infection and its epidemiology is undoubtedly important, but the fact that most infections are asymptomatic means that the impact of any education programme is going to be limited. Similarly, whilst advice about decreasing the exposure risk should always be given its impact too is likely to be small. The issues of screening for neonatal herpes and the use of suppressive acyclovir therapy have been discussed in the previous section. Here as well, it is unlikely that these approaches will markedly decrease the total number of individuals who develop clinical herpes.

Theoretically the development of a vaccine or vaccines to prevent herpes is an exciting prospect but it does pose a number of interesting issues. Can a vaccine be produced which is safe and prevents both the development of clinical herpes and the establishment of latency? As discussed in Chap. 2, HSV may be involved in the development of cervical cancer and consequently any vaccine evaluated in humans should not contain viral DNA. The development of subunit vaccines (discussed below) seems to overcome this issue.

What of immunogenicity? Antibodies are produced to a large number of viral products including proteins and glycoproteins, but which of these (if any) is involved in the production of protective immunity remains unknown (see Chap. 1). One theoretical consideration that should not be forgotten is that a vaccine may increase the likelihood of the establishment of latency thereby increasing the pool of *latently* infected individuals rather than decreasing it.

Types of HSV Vaccine

Several types of vaccine have been produced. These include live attenuated (Price et al. 1975; Scriba 1978), killed whole virus (Nasemann and Wassilew 1979; Anderson and Kilbourne 1961), and various "subunit" vaccines (Klein et al. 1981; Thompson et al. 1981; Skinner et al. 1980; Hilleman et al. 1981). The latter include purification of subunit preparations, by affinity chromatography (Long et al. 1985; Chan 1983) or a variety of other purification and extraction techniques (Meignier 1985),development of synthetic peptides (Eisenberg et al. 1985), and cloning of glycoprotein genes into expression vectors to produce large quantities of purified proteins (Watson and Enquist 1985; Lasky et al. 1984). This last group will be considered under the heading of Live vaccines, below. The theoretical advantages of each of these are summarised in Table 8.3.

Table 8.3. Suggested vaccines for herpes simplex infections

Vaccines	Comment
Live vaccines	
Unattenuated HSV	Ineffective unsafe abandoned
Attenuated HSV Deletion mutants	Safety and efficacy unknown
Heterologous herpes viruses Bovine mamilitis virus TK negative marmoset herpesvirus	Concerns re. safety
Vaccinia with cloned HSV glycoprotein genes	See the text
Inactivated vaccines Whole virus	Concerns re. safety of HSV DNA
Subunit vaccines Purified polypeptides and glycoproteins	Variable efficacy in animal experiments
Synthetic polypeptides	Human safety and efficacy unknown
Anti–idiotype antibodies	See the text

Live Vaccines

HSV produces an immune response (see Chap. 1) and previous exposure to HSV 1 attenuates the severity of the first attack on subsequent exposure to HSV 2 (Corey and Holmes 1983; see also Chap. 4). Several small, uncontrolled reports have suggested that inoculation of live virus may decrease the severity and frequency of recurrences in patients with established recurrent muco-cutaneous herpes (Macher 1957; Goldman 1961; Panscharewski and Rhode 1957), whereas other authors have reported that autoinoculation has lead to repeated HSV recurrences at the inoculation site (Lazar 1956; Blank and Haines 1973). Not surprisingly, such procedures have now been abandoned.

Viral mutants with attenuated virulence have long been known to occur spontaneously (Levaditi 1926) but because their genetic stability cannot be guaranteed (Kaerner et al. 1983; Thompson and Stevens 1983), and there is difficulty in anticipating how far biological properties such as latency and virulence are affected, such spontaneously occurring mutants have not been evaluated for vaccines.

The major objective in producing a genetically engineered live HSV vaccine is to produce viruses with the ability to replicate but with the sequences responsible for latency, neurovirulence (they may well be related) and oncogenesis either removed or deleted. The techniques involved in the production of such vaccines have been reviewed (Meignier 1985). A number of deletion mutants have been produced (Meignier 1985; Roizman and Arsenakis 1985; Mocarski et al. 1980; Post et al. 1981; Post and Roizman 1981). They appear to be genetically stable and have their virulence attenuated and some appear to prevent the development of latency. Their oncogenic potential has not been evaluated.

Two other approaches have been suggested for a live vaccine. The first of these is the use of a heterologous herpes virus; such an approach has been used in Marek's disease, where a herpes virus from turkeys prevents Marek's disease developing in chickens. Bovine mammillitis virus (Skinner et al. 1987) and a TK-negative marmoset herpes virus deletion mutant (Kit et al. 1983) have both been suggested as potential candidates for a human vaccine but safety concerns are likely to limit their potential use.

The most exciting prospect on the live vaccine front involves the cloning of HSV glycoprotein genes into an unrelated vector, such as vaccinia. There are two theoretical problems with this approach. The first is that the immunogenicity of such a vaccine may be impaired because large sections of the population had already been exposed to the vaccinia, and secondly the first use of such a campaign may impair the potential future use of this method with other immunogens (Meignier 1985). The latter problem could be overcome by insertion of several genes into the large vaccinia genome, thus creating a recombinant able to protect against several infectious agents (e.g. HIV, human papilloma virus, HSV 1, HSV 2 and hepatitis B).

It should not be forgotten also that the World Health Organization recommended stopping the use of vaccinia after the eradication of smallpox in 1976 because of the severe post-vaccination incidents (Arita and Fenner 1985).

Vaccinia virus recombinants have been constructed and tested in animals (Paoletti and Panicali 1984; Cremer et al. 1985). These vaccines offer excellent protection against lethal infection with both HSV 1 and 2 in mice and also prevent latency. Further experiments, particularly with inserts of genes against several viruses are awaited with interest.

Inactivated Whole-Virus Vaccines

Inactivated whole-virus vaccines were widely used in many parts of the world from the late 1940s until the mid 1970s. There is an extensive literature on the subject which has been reviewed (Meignier 1985). These vaccines were mostly used not to prevent herpes infection but to alleviate recurrences in patients with established recurrent herpes – so-called vaccinotherapy. Because of the theoretical risk of oncogenesis related to HSV DNA, these vaccines have largely been discontinued.

Subunit Vaccines

Extensive studies in animals have been conducted with subunit preparations derived by a variety of extraction and purification techniques. The methods used for the production of these mixtures of viral polypeptides and glycoproteins have been reviewed (Meignier 1985). The majority of the animal experiments in mice, guinea pigs and rabbits show that these vaccines are immunogenic, that they decrease mortality and morbidity on subsequent challenge and may prevent the establishment of latency (Kitces et al. 1977; Kutinova et al. 1980; Slichtova et al. 1980; Klein et al. 1981; Thornton et al. 1982; Cappel et al. 1979; Carter et al. 1981; Thompson et al. 1983; Long et al. 1985; Chan 1983). In order to produce immunity these vaccines may require repeated injections and the use of adjuvants.

Several of the subunit vaccines have been tested in humans. The efficacy of these cannot be determined, as none has been tested in randomised, double-blind placebo-controlled studies (Skinner et al. 1982a, b; Woodman et al. 1983; Cappel et al. 1985; Ashley and Corey 1983). These vaccines do appear to produce an antibody response but whether this is protective or not remains to be determined.

Synthetic polypeptides to HSV 1 and 2 gD have been produced (Eisenberg et al. 1985). Whilst not immunogenic alone, when coupled with a carrier protein (keyhole limpet haemocyanin) and adjuvant they produce a neutralising antibody response. A number of difficulties still remain with this technique including the fact that intact glycoproteins offer a greater degree of protection than synthetic polypeptides, and the effect on latency has not yet been studied.

One final new idea is worthy of mention, the possible development of an anti-herpes vaccine involving the use of anti-idiotype antibodies. These antibodies are specific for determinants (idiotypes) on the heavy or light immunoglobulin chains. Anti-idiotype antibodies can mimic the biological function of antigens (e.g. anti-idiotype induced by immunisation with anti-insulin antibodies mimics the function of insulin; Sege and Peterson 1978). This technique has already demonstrated antiviral immunity to several viruses including hepatitis B (Kennedy and Dreesman 1984), rabies (Reagan et al. 1985), Sendai virus (Ertl and Finberg 1984), reovirus (Sharpe et al. 1984), and poliovirus (Uytdehaag and Osterhaus 1985).

Future Prospects

The possible production of a safe, immunogenic vaccine, not containing DNA and able to protect against clinical illness and the development of latency, still seems to be some way off. Yet despite all the previous problems, the state of knowledge of molecular virology and the numerous new and exciting ideas may still bear fruit. Having produced a vaccine that fulfills all the criteria outlined above, the researcher will need to establish its efficacy in carefully conducted, randomised, placebo-controlled trials. This may well prove to be the most difficult part of the entire operation.

References

Adler MW, Mindel A (1983) Genital herpes – hype or hope. Br Med J 286: 1767–1768

Adler MW, Mindel A (1985) Genital infection. Antiviral Chemotherapy and Interpheron. Br Med Bull 41: 361–366

Anderson WA, Kilbourne ED (1961) Immunisation of mice with inactivated herpes simplex virus. Proc Soc Exp Biol Med 107: 518–520

Andrews EB, Tilson HH, Hurn BAL, Cordero JF and the Acyclovir in Pregnancy Advisory Committee (1988) Acyclovir in Pregnancy Registry: an observational epidemiologic approach. Am J Med 85 [suppl 2A]: 123–128

Arita I, Fenner F (1985) Complicators of smallpox vaccination. In: Quinnan GU Jr (ed). Vaccinia viruses as vectors for vaccine antigens. Elsevier, New York pp 48–60

Ashley RL, Corey L (1983) Development of antibodies to a herpes simplex virus type 2 (HSV 2) subunit vaccine in seropositive and seronegative volunteers. In: Abstracts of papers presented at an international herpes virus workshop, p 262

Bauer DJ (1977) The specific treatment of virus disease. University Park Press, Baltimore, OH.

Belsey EM, Adler MW (1978) Current approaches to the diagnosis of herpes genitalis. Br J Vener Dis 54: 115–117

Binkin NJ, Koplan JP, Cates W (1984) Preventing neonatal herpes. The value of weekly viral cultures in pregnant women with recurrent genital herpes. JAMA 251: 2816–2821

Blank H, Haines HG (1973) Experimental human reinfection with herpes simplex virus. J Invest Dermatol 61: 223–225

Bodey GP, Gottlieb J, McCredie KB, Freireich EJ (1975) Adenine arabinoside in cancer chemotherapy. In: Pavan-Langston D, Buchanan RA, Alford CA, Jr (eds) Adenine arabinoside: an antiviral agent. Raven Press, New York pp 281–285

Bouffat P, Saurat JH (1980) Isoprinosine as a therapeutic agent in recurrent mucocutaneous infections due to herpes virus. Int J Immunopharmacol 2: Abstract.

Brigden D (1985) Skin infections. Antiviral chemotherapy and interferon. Br Med Bull 41: 357–360

Brown ZA, Vontver LA, Benedetti J et al (1987) Effects on Infants of a first episode of genital herpes during pregnancy. N Engl J Med 317: 1246–1251

Bryson YJ, Dillon M, Lovett M et al. (1983) Treatment of first episodes of genital herpes simplex virus infection with oral acyclovir. N Engl J Med 308: 916–921

Buchanan RA, Hess F (1980) Vidarabine (ViraA) pharmacology and clinical experience. Pharmacol Ther 8: 143–171

Burns WH, Saral R, Santos GW, et al. (1982) Isolation and characterisation of resistant herpes simplex virus after acyclovir therapy. Lancet i: 421–423

Cappel R, De Cuyper F, De Braekeeler J (1979) Antibody and cell mediated immunity to a DNA free herpes simplex subunit vaccine. Dev Biol Stand 43: 381–385

Cappel R, Sprecher S, De Cuyper F, De Braekeleer J (1985) Clinical efficacy of a herpes simplex subunit vaccine. J Med Virol 16: 137–145

Carter CA, Hartley CE, Skinner GRB, Turner SP, Easty DL (1981) Experimental ulcerative herpetic keratitis. IV. Preliminary observations on the efficacy of a herpes simplex subunit vaccine. Br J Ophthalmol 65: 679–682

Chan WL (1983) Protective immunisation of mice with specific HSV 1 glycoproteins. Immunology 49: 343–352

Cheng YC, Dutschman G, Fox JJ, Watanabe KA, Machida H (1981) Differential activity of potential antiviral nucleoside analogs on herpes simplex virus-induced and human cellular thymidine kinases. Antimicrob Agents Chemother 20: 420–423

Chou S, Gallagher JG, Merigan TC (1981) Controlled clinical trial of intravenous acyclovir in heart-transplant patients with mucocutaneous herpes simplex infections. Lancet i: 1392–1394

Coen CM, Schaffer PA (1981) Two distinct loci confer resistance to acycloguanosine in herpes simplex virus type 1. Proc Natl Acad Sci USA 77: 2265–2269

Colin J, Tournoux A, Chastel C, Reynard G (1981) Superficial herpes simplex keratitis. Double blind comparative trial of acyclovir and idoxuridine. Nouv Press Méd 10: 2969–2975

Collum LMT, Benedict-Smith A, Hilary IB (1980) Randomised double blind trial of acyclovir and idoxuridine in dendritic corneal ulceration. Br J Ophthalmol 64: 766–769

Collum LMT, Logan P, Ravenscroft T (1983) Acyclovir (Zovirax) in herpetic disciform keratitis. Br J Ophthalmol 67: 115–118

Committee on Fetus and Newborn (1980) Perinatal herpes simplex virus infections. Pediatrics 66: 147–148

Corey L (1985) Genital Herpes. In: Holmes KK, Mårdh P-A, Sparling PF, Wiesner PJ (eds) Sexually transmitted diseases. McGraw-Hill Book Company, New York pp 449–474

Corey L (1986) Genital herpes simplex virus infections: natural history and therapy. In: Oriel J D, Harris JRW (eds) Recent advances in sexually transmitted diseases, vol 3, Churchill Livingstone, Edinburgh, pp 71–108

Corey L, Holmes KK (1983) Genital herpes simplex virus infections: current concepts in diagnosis, therapy and prevention. Ann Intern Med 98: 973–983

Corey L, Spear PG (1986) Infections with herpes simplex viruses. (Second of two parts.) N Engl J Med 314: 749–757

Corey L, Reeves WC, Chiang WT et al. (1978) Ineffectiveness of topical ether for the treatment of herpes simplex virus infection. N Engl J Med 299: 237–239

Corey L, Chiang WT, Reeves WC, Stamm WE, Brewar L, Holmes KK (1979) Effect of isoprinosine on the cellular immune response in initial genital herpes virus infection. Clin Res 27: 41A

Corey L, Nahmias AJ, Guinan ME, Benedetti JK, Critchlow CW, Holmes KK (1982) A trial of topical acyclovir in genital herpes virus infections. N Engl J Med 306: 1313–1319

Corey L, Fife KH, Benedetti JK et al (1983) Intravenous acyclovir for the treatment of primary genital herpes. Ann Intern Med 98: 914–921

Corey L, Mindel A, Fife KH, Sutherland S, Benedetti J, Adler MW (1985) Risk of recurrence after treatment of first episode genital herpes with intravenous acyclovir. Sex Transm Dis 12: 215–218

Corey LC, Whitley RJ, Stone EF, Mohan K (1988) Difference between herpes simplex virus type 1 and type 2 neonatal encephalitis in neurological outcome. Lancet i: 1–4

Coster DJ, Jones BR, McGill J (1979) Treatment of amoeboid herpetic ulcers with adenine arabinoside or trifluorothymidine. Br J Ophthalmol 63: 418–421

Coster DJ, Wilhelmus KR, Michaud R, Jones BR (1983) A comparison of acyclovir and idoxuridine in treatment for ulcerative herpetic keratitis. Br J Ophthalmol 95: 175–181

Cremer KJ, Mackett M, Wohlenberg C, Notkins AL, Moss B (1985) Vaccinia virus recombinant expressing herpes simplex virus type 1 glycoprotein D prevents latent herpes in mice. Science 228: 737–740

Crumpacker CS, Schnipper LE, Marlow SI, Kowalsky PN, Hershey BJ, Levin MJ (1982) Resistance to antiviral drugs of herpes simplex virus isolated from a patient treated with acyclovir. N Engl J Med 306: 343–346

Csonka GW, Tyrrell DAJ (1984) Treatment of herpes genitalis with carbenoxolone and cicloxolone cream: a double blind placebo controlled clinical trial. Br J Vener Dis 60: 178–181

Dargan DJ, Subak-Sharpe JH (1986) The antiviral activity against herpes simplex virus of the triterpenoid compounds carbenoxolone sodium and cicloxolone sodium. J Antimicrob Chemother 18 [suppl B]: 185–200.

Dawson CR (1984) Ocular herpes simplex virus infections. Clin Dermatol 2: 56–66

De Clercq E (1985) Recent trends and development in antiviral chemotherapy. In Proceedings of the First International TNO Conference on Antiviral Research; Rotterdam. Antiviral Res [Suppl 1]: 11–19

De Clercq E, Descamps J, De Somer P, Barr PJ, Jones AS, Walker RT (1979) (E)-5-(2-bromovinyl)-2′-deoxyuridine: a potent and selective anti-herpes agent. Proc Natl Acad Sci USA 76: 2947–2951

Derman RJ (1986) Counselling the herpes genitalis patient. J Reprod Med 31 [suppl]: 439–444

Douglas JM, Critchlow C, Benedetti J et al. (1984) A double blind study of oral acyclovir for suppression of recurrences of genital herpes simplex virus infection. N Engl J Med 310: 1551–1556

Eisenberg JR, Cerini PC, Heilman CJ, et al (1985) Synthetic glycoprotein D-related peptides protect mice against herpes simplex virus challenge. J Virol 56: 1014–1017

Elion GB (1982) Mechanism of action and selectivity of acyclovir. Am J Med 73 [suppl 1A]: 7–13

Ertl HCJ, Finberg RW (1984) Sendai virus-specific T-cell clones: induction of cytolytic T cells by an anti-idiotype antibody directed against a helper T-cell clone. Proc Natl Acad Sci USA 81: 2850–2854

Farrell RG, Nesland RS (1977) Topical ethyl ether therapy of herpes simplex infections. J Am Coll Emerg Physic 6: 372–373

Fawcett HA, Wansbrough-Jones MH, Clark AE, Leigh IM (1983) Prophylactic topical acyclovir for frequent recurrent herpes simplex infection with and without erythema multiforme. Br Med J 287: 98–99

Field HJ, Darby G, Wildy P (1980) Isolation and characterization of acyclovir-resistant mutants of herpes simplex virus. J Gen Virol 49: 115–124

Fiddian AP, Ivanyi L (1983) Topical acyclovir in the management of recurrent herpes labialis. Br J Dermatol 109: 321–326

Fiddian AP, Yeo JM, Stubbings R, Dean D (1983a) Successful treatment of herpes labialis with topical acyclovir. Br J Med 286: 1699–1700

Fiddian AP, Kinghorn GR, Golmeier D et al. (1983b) Topical acyclovir in the treatment of genital herpes: a comparison with systemic therapy. J Antimicrob Chemother. 12 [suppl B]: 67–77

Furman PA, St Clair MH, Fyfe JA, Rideout JL, Keller PM, Elion GB (1979) Inhibition of herpes simplex virus induced DNA polymerase activity and viral DNA replication by 9–(2–hydroxyethoxymethyl)guanine and its triphosphate. J Med Virol 32: 72–77

Fyfe JA (1982) Differential phosphorylation of (E)–5–(2–bromovinyl–2'–deoxyuridine monophosphate by thymidylate kinases from herpes simplex viruses types 1 and 2 and varicella zoster virus. Mol Pharmacol 21: 432–437

Galli M, Lazzarin A, Moroni M, Zanussi C (1982) Inosiplex in recurrent herpes simplex infections. Lancet ii: 331–332

Gaub J, Pedersen C, Poulson A-G, et al (1987) The effect of Foscarnet (phosphonoformate) on human immunodeficiency virus isolation, T-cell subsets and lymphocyte function in AIDS patients. AIDS 1: 27–33

Glezerman M, Lunenfeld E, Cohen V, et al. (1988) Placebo-controlled trial of topical interferon in labial and genital herpes. Lancet i: 150–152

Gold D, Benedetti J, Corey L (1986) Topical surfactant therapy for recurrent herpes simplex infection. Lancet ii: 283

Goldberg CB (1986) Controlled trial of "Intervir-A" in herpes simplex virus infection. Lancet i: 703–706

Goldman L (1961) Reactions of an auto inoculation for recurrent herpes simplex. Arch Dermatol 84: 1025–1026

Halsos AM, Salo OP, Lassus A, et al. (1985) Oral acyclovir suppression of recurrent genital herpes: a double-blind, placebo controlled cross-over study. Acta Derm Venereol (Stockh) 65: 59–63

Hann IM, Prentice HG, Blacklock HA, et al (1983) Acyclovir prophylaxis against herpes virus infection in severely immunocompromised patients: randomised double blind trial. Br Med J 287: 384–388

Heidelberger C, King D (1979) Trifluorothymidine. Pharmacol Ther 6: 427–442

Herrman EC Jr (1961) Plaque inhibition test for detection of specific inhibitors of DNA containing viruses. Proc Soc Exp Biol Med 107: 142–145

Hilleman MR, Larson VH, Lehman ED, et al (1981) Sub-unit herpes simplex virus-2 vaccines In: Nahmias AJ, Dowdle WR, Schinazi RF (eds) The human herpesviruses. Elsevier, New York, pp 503–506

Huang ES, Huang CH, Huong SM, Selgrade M (1976) Preferential inhibition of herpes group viruses by phosphonoacetic acid: effect on virus DNA synthesis and virus-induced DNA polymerase activity. Yale J Biol Med 49: 93–98

Jones BR, Coster DJ, Falcon MG, Cantell K (1976) Topical therapy of ulcerative herpetic keratitis with human interferon. Lancet ii: 128

Kaerner HC, Schroder CH, Ott-Hartmann A, Kummel G, Kircher H (1983) Genetic variability of herpes simplex virus: development of a pathogenic variant during passaging of a non-pathogenic herpes simplex virus type 1 virus strain in mouse brain. J Virol 46: 83–93

Kennedy RC, Dreesman GR (1984) Enhancement of the immune response to hepatitis B surface antigen. In vivo administration of anti-idiotype induces anti-HBs that express a similar idiotype. J Exp Med 159: 655–665

Kinghorn GR, Turner EB, Barton IG, Potter CW, Burke CA, Fiddian AP (1983) Efficacy of topical acyclovir cream in first and recurrent episodes of genital herpes. Antiviral Res 3: 291–301

Kinghorn GR, Jeavons M, Rowland M et al. (1985) Acyclovir prophylaxis of recurrent genital herpes: a randomised placebo controlled crossover study. Genitourin Med 61: 387–390

Kit S, Quavi H, Dubbs DR, Otsuka H (1983) Attenuated marmoset herpes virus isolated from recombinants of virulent marmoset herpes virus and hybrid plasmids. J Med Virol 12: 25–36

Kitces EN, Morahan PS, Tew JG, Murray BK (1977) Protection from oral herpes simplex virus infection by a nucleic acid-free virus vaccine. Infect Immun 16: 955–960

Klein RJ, Buimovici-Klein E, Mosur H, Moucha R, Hilfenhaus J (1981) Efficacy of a virion envelope herpes simplex virus against experimental skin infections in hairless mice. Arch Virol 68: 73–80

Kutinova L, Vonka V, Stichtova V (1980) Immunogenicity of subviral herpes simplex virus preparations: protection of mice against intraperitoneal infection with live virus. Acta Virol (English Edition) 24: 391–398

La Lau C, Oosterhuis JA, Versteeg J, et al. (1982) Acyclovir and trifluorothymidine in herpetic keratitis: a multicentre trial. Br J Opthalmol 66: 506–508

Lasky LA, Dowbenko D, Simonson C, Berman PW (1984) Production of an HSV subunit vaccine by genetically engineered mammalian cell lines. In: Chanock RM, Lerner RA (eds) Modern approaches to vaccines: molecular and chemical basis of virus virulence and immunogenicity. Cold Spring Harbor Laboratory Press, Cold Spring Harbor, NY pp 189–194

Lazar MP (1956) Vaccination for recurrent herpes simplex infection: initiation of a new disease site following the use of unmodified material containing the live virus. Arch Dermatol 73: 70–71

Lee FK, Coleman RM, Pereira L, Bailey PD, Tatsuno M, Nahmias AJ (1985) Detection of herpes simplex virus type 2-specific antibody with glycoprotein G. J Clin Microbiol 22: 641–644

Lee FK, Pereira L, Griffin C, Reid E, Nahmias A (1986) A novel glycoprotein for detection of herpes simplex virus type 1 specific antibodies. J Virol Methods 14: 111–118

Leigh IM (1988) The management of nongenital herpes simplex virus infection in immunocompetent patients. Am J Med 85 [suppl 2A]: 34–38

Levaditi C (1926) L'herpes et le zona. Masson, Paris.

Long D, Madara TJ, Ponce de Leon M, Cohen GH, Montgomery PC, Eisenberg RJ (1985) Glycoprotein D protects mice against lethal challenge with herpes simplex virus types 1 and 2. Infect Immun 43: 761–764

Macher E (1957) Zur Behandlung des chronisch-rezivienrenden herpes simplex. Z Hautkr 23: 18–22

Mao JCH, Robishaw EE (1975) Mode of inhibition of herpes simplex virus DNA polymerase by phosphonoacetate. Biochemistry 14: 5475–5479

McCulley JP, Binder PS, Kaufman HE, O'Day DM, Poirier RH (1982) A double blind multicenter clinical trial of acyclovir vs idoxuridine for treatment of epithelial herpes simplex keratitis. Opthalmology 89: 1195–1200

McGill JI (1984) Antiviral treatment of herpes simplex stroma disease. In: Maudgal P (ed) Herpetic eye disease. Junk, Berlin pp 217–221

McGill J, Scott GM (1985) Viral keratitis. Br Med Bull 41: 351–356

McGill J, Tormey P, Walker CD (1981) Comparative trial of acyclovir and adenine arabinoside in the treatment of herpes simplex corneal ulcers. Br J Opthalmol 65: 610–613

McClaren C, Corey L, Dekker C, Barry DW (1983) In vitro sensitivity to acyclovir in genital herpes simplex viruses from acyclovir treated patients. J Infect Dis 148: 868–875

Meignier B (1985) Vaccination against herpes simplex virus infections. In: Roizman B, Lopez C (eds) The herpes viruses, vol 4, Plenum Press, New York pp 265–296

Mertz GJ, Critchlow CW, Benedetti J, et al (1984) Double blind placebo controlled trial of oral acyclovir in first episode genital herpes simplex virus infection. JAMA 252: 1147–1151

Mertz GJ, Jones CC, Mills J et al (1988) Long-term acyclovir suppression of frequently recurring genital herpes simplex virus infection. A multicenter double-blind trial. JAMA 260: 201–266

Meyers JD, Wade JC, Mitchell CD, et al. (1982) Multicenter collaborative trial of intravenous acyclovir for treatment of mucocutaneous herpes simplex virus infection in the immunocompromised host. Am J Med 73: 229–235

Meyrick Thomas RH, Dodd HJ, Yeo JM, Kirby JP (1985) Oral acyclovir in the suppression of recurrent non-genital herpes simplex virus infection. Br J Dermatol 113: 731–735

Miller WH, Miller RL (1980) Phosphorylation of acyclovir (acycloguanosine) monophosphate by GMP kinase. J Bio Chem 255: 7204-7207

Mindel A (1984) Treatment and prevention of herpes genital infection. J Antimicrob Chemother 14 [suppl A]: 75–83

Mindel A, Carney O (1988) Acyclovir malabsorption. Br Med J 296: 1605

Mindel A, Sutherland S (1983) Genital herpes – the disease and its treatment including intravenous acyclovir. J Antimicrob Chemother 12 [suppl B]: 51–59

Mindel A, Adler MW, Sutherland S, Fiddian AP (1982) Intravenous acyclovir treatment for primary genital herpes. Lancet i: 697–700

Mindel A, Weller IVD, Faherty A, et al. (1984) Prophylactic oral acyclovir in recurrent genital herpes. Lancet ii: 57–59

Mindel A, Weller IVD, Faherty A, Sutherland S, Fiddian AP, Adler MW (1986) Acyclovir in first attacks of genital herpes and prevention of recurrences. Genitourin Med 62: 28–32

Mindel A, Kinghorn G, Allason-Jones E, et al. (1987) Treatment of first-attack genital herpes acyclovir versus inosine pranobex. Lancet i: 1171–1173

Mindel A, Faherty A, Carney O, Patou G, Williams P (1988) The efficacy, dosage and safety of longterm suppressive acyclovir for the treatment of recurrent genital herpes. Lancet i: 926–928

Mindel A, Carney O, Sonnex C, Freris M, Patou G, William P (1989) Suppression of frequently recurring genital herpes. Acyclovir versus inosine pranobex. Genitourin Med 65: 103–105

Mitchell CD, Bean B, Gentry SR, Groth KE, Boen JR, Balfour HH (1981) Acyclovir therapy for mucocutaneous herpes simplex infections in immunocompromised patients. Lancet i: 1389–1392

Mocarski ES, Post LE, Roizman B (1980) Molecular engineering of the herpes simplex virus genome: insertion of a second L–S junction into the genome causes additional genome inversion. Cell 22: 243–255

Muller WEG (1977) Rational design of arabinosyl nucleosides as antitumor and antiviral agents. Jpn J Antibiot 30 [suppl]: S104–S120

Muller WEG (1979) Mechanism of action and pharmacology: chemical agents. In: Galasso G J, Merigan TC, Buchanan RA (eds) Antiviral agents and viral diseases of man. 1st edn, Raven Press, New York, pp 77–149

Nahmias AJ, Keyserling HL (1984) Neonatal herpes simplex in context of the Torch complex. In: Holmes KK, Mårdh P, Sparling PF, Wiesner PJ (eds) Sexually transmitted diseases. McGraw-Hill Book Company, New York, pp 816–826

Nahmias AJ, Josey WE, Naib ZM, Freeman MG, Fernandez RJ, Wheeler JH (1971) Perinatal risk associated with maternal genital herpes simplex virus infection. Am J Obstet Gynecol 110: 825–837

Nasemann TH, Wassilew SW (1979) Vaccination for herpes simplex genitalis. Br J Vener Dis 55: 121–122

Nilsen AE, Aasen T, Halsos AM et al. (1982) Efficacy of oral acyclovir in the treatment of initial and recurrent genital herpes. Lancet ii: 571–573

Öberg B (1983) Antiviral effects of phosphonoformate (PFA, Foscarnet sodium). Pharmacol Ther 19: 387–415

Overall JC Jr (1984) Dermatologic viral diseases. In: Galasso GJ, Merigan TC, Buchanan RA (eds) Antiviral agents and viral diseases of man, 2nd edn, Raven Press, New York, pp 247–312

Panscherewski D, Rhode B (1957) Zur Serologie und Therapie des Herpes Simplex recidivans. Hautarzt 13: 275–278

Paoletti E, Panicali D (1984) Genetically engineered pox viruses as live recombinant vaccines. In: Chanock RM and Lerner RA (eds) Modern approaches to vaccines – molecular and chemical basis of virus virulence and immunospecificity. Cold Spring Harbor Laboratory Press, Cold Spring Harbor, NY, pp 295–299

Partridge M, Poswillo DE (1984) Topical carbonoxolone sodium in the management of herpes simplex infections. Br J Oral Maxillofac Surg 22: 138–145

Patterson A, Jones BR (1967) The management of ocular herpes. Trans Opthalmol Soc UK 87: 59–84

Pavan-Langston D (1984) Ocular viral diseases. In: Galasso GJ, Merigan TC, Buchanan RA (eds) Antiviral agents and viral diseases of man, 2nd edn. Raven Press, New York, pp 207–245

Pazin GJ, Harger JH (1986) Management of oral and genital herpes simplex virus infection: diagnosis and treatment. DM 32: 725–824

Post LE, Roizman B (1981) A generalised technique for deletion of specific genes in large genomes: alpha gene 22 of herpes simplex virus 1 is not essential for growth in cell culture. Cell 25: 227–232

Post LE, Mackem S, Roizman B (1981) The regulation of alpha genes of herpes simplex virus: expression of chimeric genes produced by fusion of thymidine kinase with α gene promoters. Cell 34: 555–556

Poswillo DE, Roberts GJ (1981) Topical carbonoxolone for orofacial herpes simplex infection. Lancet ii: 143–144

Price RW, Walz MA, Wohlenberg C, Notkins AL (1975) Latent infection of sensory ganglia with herpes simplex virus: efficacy of immunisation. Science 188: 938–940

Prober CG, Sullender WM, Yasukawa LL, Au DS, Yeager AA, Arvin AM (1987) Low risk of herpes simplex virus infections in neonates exposed to the virus at the time of vaginal delivery to mothers with recurrent genital herpes simplex virus infection. N Engl J Med 316: 240–244

Prusoff WH (1959) Synthesis and biological activities of iododeoxyuridine, an analog of thymidine. Biochem Biophys Acta 132: 295–296

Prusoff WH, Goz B (1975) Halogenated pyrimidine deoxyribonucleosides. In: Eichler O, Herken F H, Welch AD (eds) Handbook of experimental pharmacology, vol 38, part 2. Springer, Berlin, Heidelberg, New York, pp 272–347

Prusoff WH, Ward DC (1976) Commentary: nucleosides analogs with antiviral activity. Biochem Pharmacol 25: 1233–1239

Prusoff WH, Chen MS, Fischer PH, et al. (1979) Antiviral iodinated pyrimidine deoxyribonucleosides: 5–iodo–2'–deoxyuridine; 5–iodo–2'–deoxycytidine; 5–iodo–5'–amino–2',5'–dideoxyuridine. Pharmacol Ther 7: 1–34

Raborn GW, McGaw WT, Grace M, Percy J (1988) Treatment of herpes labialis with acyclovir: review of three clinical trials. Am J Med 85 [suppl 2A]: 39–42

Reagan KJ, Wunner WH, Koprowski H (1985) Viral antigen-independent immunization: induction by anti-idiotypic antibodies of neutralizing antibodies to defined epitopes on rabies virus glycoprotein,. In: Dreesman GR, Bronson JG, Kennedy RC (eds) High technology route to virus vaccines. Am Soc Microbiol, Washington DC, pp 117–124

Reichman RC, Badger GJ, Mertz GJ, et al. (1984) Treatment of recurrent genital herpes simplex infection with oral acyclovir: a controlled trial. JAMA 251: 2103–2107

Roizman B, Arsenakis M (1985) Genetic engineering of herpes simplex virus genomes for attentuation and expression of foreign genes. In: Quinnan G U Jr (ed). Vaccinia viruses as vectors for vaccine antigens. Elsevier, New York, pp 211–223

Sacks SL, Portnoy J, Lawee D et al. (1987) Clinical course of recurrent genital herpes and treatment with Foscarnet cream: results of a Canadian multicenter trial. J Infect Dis 155: 178–186

Salo O, Lassus A (1983) Treatment of recurrent genital herpes with isoprinosine. Eur J Sex Trans Dis 1: 101–105

Salo OP, Lassus A, Hovi R, Fiddian AP (1983) Double blind placebo controlled trial of oral acyclovir in recurrent genital herpes. Eur J Sex Trans Dis 1: 95–98

Saral R, Burns WH, Laskin OL, Santos GW, Lietman PS (1981) Acyclovir prophylaxis of herpes simplex virus infections. A randomised, double-blind, controlled trial in bone-marrow transplant recipients. N Engl J Med 305: 63–67

Saral R, Ambinder RF, Burns WH et al. (1983) Acyclovir prophylaxis against herpes simplex virus infection in patients with leukemia. Ann Intern Med 99: 773–776

Schädelin J, Schilt U, Rohner M (1988) Prevention of labialis following trigeminal surgery. Am J Med 85 [suppl 2A]: 46–48

Schinazi RF, Del Bene V, Taylor Scott R, Dudley-Thorpe J (1986) Characterisation of acyclovir resistant and sensitive herpes simplex viruses isolated from a patient with an acquired immune deficiency. J Antimicrob Chemother 18 [suppl B]: 127–134

Schnipper LE, Crumpacker CS (1980) Resistance of herpes simplex virus to acycloguanosine: role of viral thymidine kinase and DNA polymerase loci. Proc Natl Acad Sci USA 77: 2270–2273

Scriba M (1978) Protection of guinea pigs against primary and recurrent genital herpes infection by immunization with live heterologous or homologous herpes simplex virus: implication for a herpes virus vaccine. Med Microbiol Immunol 166: 63–69

Sege K, Peterson PA (1978) Use of anti-idiotypic antibodies as cell surface receptor probes. Proc Natl Acad Sci USA 75: 2443–2447

Sharpe AH, Gaulton GN, McDade KK, Fields BN, Greene MI (1984) Syngeneic monoclonal antiidiotype can induce cellular immunity to reovirus. J Exp Med 160: 1195–1205

Shaw M, King M, Best JM, Banatvala JE, Gibson JR, Klaber MR (1985) Failure of acyclovir cream in treatment of recurrent herpes labialis. Br Med J 291: 7–9

Sibrack CD, Gutman LT, Wilfert CM, et al. (1982) Pathogenicity of acyclovir-resistant herpes simplex virus type 1 from an immunodeficient child. J Infect Dis 146: 673–682

Skinner G, Buchan A, Hartley CE, Turner SP, William DR (1980) The preparation, efficacy and safety of "antigenoid" vaccine NFU(S⁻L⁺) MRC towards prevention of herpes simplex virus infections in human subjects. Med Microbiol Immunol 169: 39–51

Skinner GRB, Woodman G, Hartley CE, et al. (1982a) Early experience with "antigenoid" vaccine Ac NFU (S⁻) MRC towards prevention and modification of herpes genitalis. Dev Biol Stand 52: 333–344

Skinner GRB, Woodman GB, Hartley CE, et al. (1982b) Preparation and immunogenicity of vaccine Ac NFU (S⁻) MRC towards the prevention of herpes genitalis. Br J Vener Dis 58: 381–386

Skinner GRB, Buchan A, Durham J et al. (1987) Role of bovine mammillitis virus towards preparation of an alternative vaccine against herpes simplex virus infections of human subjects. Vaccine 5: 55–59

Sköldenberg B, Forsgren M, Alestig K, et al. (1984) Acyclovir versus vidarabine in herpes simplex encephalitis. Randomised multicentre study in consecutive Swedish patients. Lancet ii: 707–711

Slichtova V, Kutinova L, Vonka V (1980) Immunogenicity of subviral herpes virus type 1 preparation: protection of mice against intradermal challenge with type 1 and type 2 viruses. Arch Virol 66: 207–214

Spruance SL (1988) Cutaneous herpes simplex virus lesions induced by ultraviolet radiation: a review of model systems and prophylactic therapy with oral acyclovir. Am J Med 85 [suppl 2A]: 43–45

Spruance SL, Schnipper LE, Overall JC Jr, et al. (1982) Treatment of herpes simplex labialis with topical acyclovir in polyethylene glycol. J Infect Dis 146: 85–90

Straus SE, Takiff HE, Seidlin M, et al. (1984) Suppression of frequently recurring genital herpes. A placebo controlled double blind trail of oral acyclovir. N Engl J Med 316: 1545–1550

Sugar J, Kaufman HE (1973) Halogenated pyrimidines in antiviral therapy. In: Carter W A (ed) Selective inhibition of viral functions. CRC Press, Cleveland, OH, pp 295–311

Sullivan-Bolyai J, Hill HF, Wilson C, Corey L (1983) Neonatal herpes simplex virus infection in King County, Washington. Increasing incidence and epidemiologic correlates. JAMA 250: 3059–3062

Taylor CA, Hendley SO, Greer KE, Gwaltney JM (1977) Topical treatment of herpes labialis with chloroform. Arch Dermatol 113: 1550–1552

Thin RN, Nabarro JM, Davidson Parker J, Fiddian AP (1983) Topical acyclovir in the treatment of initial genital herpes. Br J Vener Dis 59: 116–119

Thin RN, Jeffries, DJ, Taylor PK, et al. (1985) Recurrent genital herpes suppressed by oral acyclovir: a multicentre double-blind trial. J Antimicrob Chemother 16: 219–226

Thompson RL, Stevens J (1983) Replication of body temperature selects a neurovirulent herpes simplex virus type 2. Infect Immun 41: 855–857

Thompson TA, Murray BK, Morahan PS, Cline P (1981) Protective studies on several herpes simplex type 1 vaccine preparations in a mouse labial infection model. In: Nahmias AJ, Dowdle WR, Schinazi RF (eds) The human herpesviruses. New York, Elsevier, pp 649–650

Thompson TA, Hilfenhaus J, Mosar H, Morahan PS (1983) Comparison of effects of adjuvants in efficacy of virion envelope herpes simplex virus vaccine against labial infection of Balb/c mice. Infect Immun 41: 556–562

Thornton B, Griffiths JB, Walkland A (1982) Herpes simplex vaccine using cell membrane associated antigen in animal models. Dev Biol Stand 50: 201–206

Uytdehaag IGCM, Osterhaus ADME (1985) Induction of neutralising antibody in mice against poliovirus type II with monoclonal anti–idiotypic antibody. J Immunol 134: 1225–1229

Van Etta L, Brown J, Mastri A, Wilson T (1981) Fatal vidarabine toxicity in a patient with normal renal function. JAMA 246: 1703–1705

Vontver LA, Reeves WC, Rattray M et al (1979) Clinical course and diagnosis of genital herpes simplex virus infection and evaluation of topical surfactant therapy. Am J Obstet Gynecol 133: 548–554

Wade C, Newton B, McLaren C, Flournoy N, Keeney RE (1982) Intravenous acyclovir to treat mucocutaneous herpes simplex virus infection after marrow transplantation. Ann Intern Med 96: 265–269

Wade JC, McLaren C, Meyers JD (1983) Frequency and significance of acyclovir-resistant herpes simplex virus isolated from marrow transplant patients receiving multiple courses treatment with acyclovir. J Infect Dis 148: 1077–1082

Wade JC, Newton B, Flournoy N, Meyers JD (1984) Oral acyclovir for prevention of herpes simplex virus reactivation after marrow transplantation. Ann Intern Med 100: 823–828

Wallin J, Lernestedt JO, Ogenstad S, Lycke E (1985) Topical treatment of recurrent genital herpes infection with Forscarnet. Scand J Infect Dis 17: 165–172

Watson RJ, Enquist L (1985) Genetically engineered herpes simplex virus vaccines. In: Melnick J L (ed) Progress in medical virology, vol 31. Karger, Basel pp. 84–108

Weller IVD, Carreño V, Fowler MJF, et al (1983) Acyclovir in hepatitis B antigen-positive chronic liver disease: inhibition of viral replication and transient renal impairment with IV bolus administration. J Antimicrob Chemother 11: 223–231

Whitley RJ (1988) Herpes simplex infection of the central nervous system. Am J Med 85 [suppl 2A]: 61–67

Whitley RJ, Ch'ien LT, Dolin R, Galasso GJ, Alford CA Editors and the collaborative study group (1976). Adenine arabinoside therapy of herpes zoster in the immunosuppressed. NIAID collaborative antiviral study. N Engl J Med 294: 1193–1199

Whitley RJ, Soong SJ, Dolin R, et al. (1977) Adenine arabinoside therapy of biopsy-proved herpes simplex virus encephalitis. National Institute of Allergy and Infectious Diseases collaborative antiviral study. N Engl J Med 297: 289–294

Whitley RJ, Tucker BC, Kinkel AW, et al. (1980a) Pharmacology, tolerance and antiviral activity of vidarabine monophosphate in humans. Antimicrob Agents Chemother 18: 709–715

Whitley RJ, Nahmias AJ, Soong SJ, Galasso GJ, Fleming CL, Alford CA (1980b) Vidarabine therapy of neonatal herpes simplex virus infection. Pediatrics 66: 495–501

Whitley RJ, Soon SJ, Linneman C, Liu C, Pazin G, Alford CA (1982) Herpes simplex encephalitis. JAMA 247: 317–320

Whitley RJ, Alford CA, Hirsch MS, et al (1986) Vidarabine versus acyclovir therapy in herpes simplex encephalitis. N Engl J Med 314: 144–149

Woodman CBJ, Buchan A, Fuller A, et al. (1983) Efficacy of a vaccine Ac NFU, (S⁻) MRC5 given after an initial clinical episode in the prevention of herpes genitalis. Br J Vener Dis 59: 311–313

Young BJ, Patterson A, Ravenscroft T (1982) A randomised double blind clinical trial of acyclovir (Zovirax) and adenine arabinoside in herpes simplex corneal ulceration. Br J Ophthalmol 66: 361–363

Subject Index